Exhibiting Health

Critical Issues in Health and Medicine

Edited by Rima D. Apple, University of Wisconsin–Madison and
Janet Golden, Rutgers University–Camden

Growing criticism of the U.S. healthcare system is coming from consumers, politicians, the media, activists, and healthcare professionals. Critical Issues in Health and Medicine is a collection of books that explores these contemporary dilemmas from a variety of perspectives, among them political, legal, historical, sociological, and comparative, and with attention to crucial dimensions such as race, gender, ethnicity, sexuality, and culture.

For a list of titles in the series, see the last page of the book

Exhibiting Health

Public Health Displays in the Progressive Era

Jennifer Lisa Koslow

Rutgers University Press

New Brunswick, Camden, and Newark, New Jersey, and London

Library of Congress Cataloging-in-Publication Data

Names: Koslow, Jennifer Lisa, 1970– author.
Title: Exhibiting health: public health displays in the progressive era / Jennifer Lisa Koslow.
Description: New Brunswick, New Jersey: Rutgers University Press, 2020. | Series: Critical
   issues in health and medicine | Includes bibliographical references and index.
Identifiers: LCCN 2019048897 | ISBN 9781978803268 (paperback) | ISBN 9781978803275
   (hardback) | ISBN 9781978803282 (epub) | ISBN 9781978803299 (mobi) |
   ISBN 9781978803305 (pdf)
Subjects: MESH: Exhibits as Topic | Health Education—history | Public Health—history |
   Communicable Disease Control | Disease Transmission,
Infectious—prevention & control | History, 20th Century | United States
Classification: LCC RA425 | NLM WA 27 | DDC 362.1—dc23
LC record available at https://lccn.loc.gov/2019048897

A British Cataloging-in-Publication record for this book is available from the British Library.

⊛ The paper used in this publication meets the requirements of the American National
Standard for Information Sciences—Permanence of Paper for Printed Library Materials,
ANSI Z39.48-1992.

www.rutgersuniversitypress.org

Manufactured in the United States of America

For Benjamin and Ramona

Contents

Exhibiting Health

Valuing the Visual in Public Health Education

In October 1913, Key West's health officer, Joseph Y. Porter Jr., sent Florida's chief health officer, Joseph Y. Porter (Porter Jr.'s father), four photographs of a fly exhibit that he had created for the benefit of the city's residents.[1] Flies were a topic of public health concern across the nation, and Key West's long history of yellow fever outbreaks meant that it was no exception. Moreover, yellow fever was a personal issue; Porter's grandparents both died of it.

Using the front porch of his office, Porter Jr. explained the various ways in which flies served as vectors of disease. He tacked up a small poster on a bench of an oversized fly titled "the world's greatest murderer THE FLY." On a crate next to the bench, Porter fastened an even larger sign in Spanish, presumably to target the island's approximately 2,600 Cuban residents.[2] Its headline read: "De Las Moscas e Inmundicias a la Comida y la Fiebre" (translation: Of flies and filth to the food and fever). He also put out two transparent gauze-covered containers with organic materials (what exactly is inside is obscured in the photographs). Although Porter designed the exhibit to be temporary, his photography permanently captured its essence. Porter intended to change individual behaviors concerning public health threats through the public's examination of living objects and related visual materials.

Porter's attempt to make exhibit engagement an ordinary aspect of popular public health education was not exceptional. Instead, it was an idea that other public health officials and health reformers replicated numerous times in the early twentieth century.[3] This is a study of the rising appeal and eventual rejection of the exhibition as a common mechanism for popular public health education, a movement that occurred roughly between 1900 and 1930.

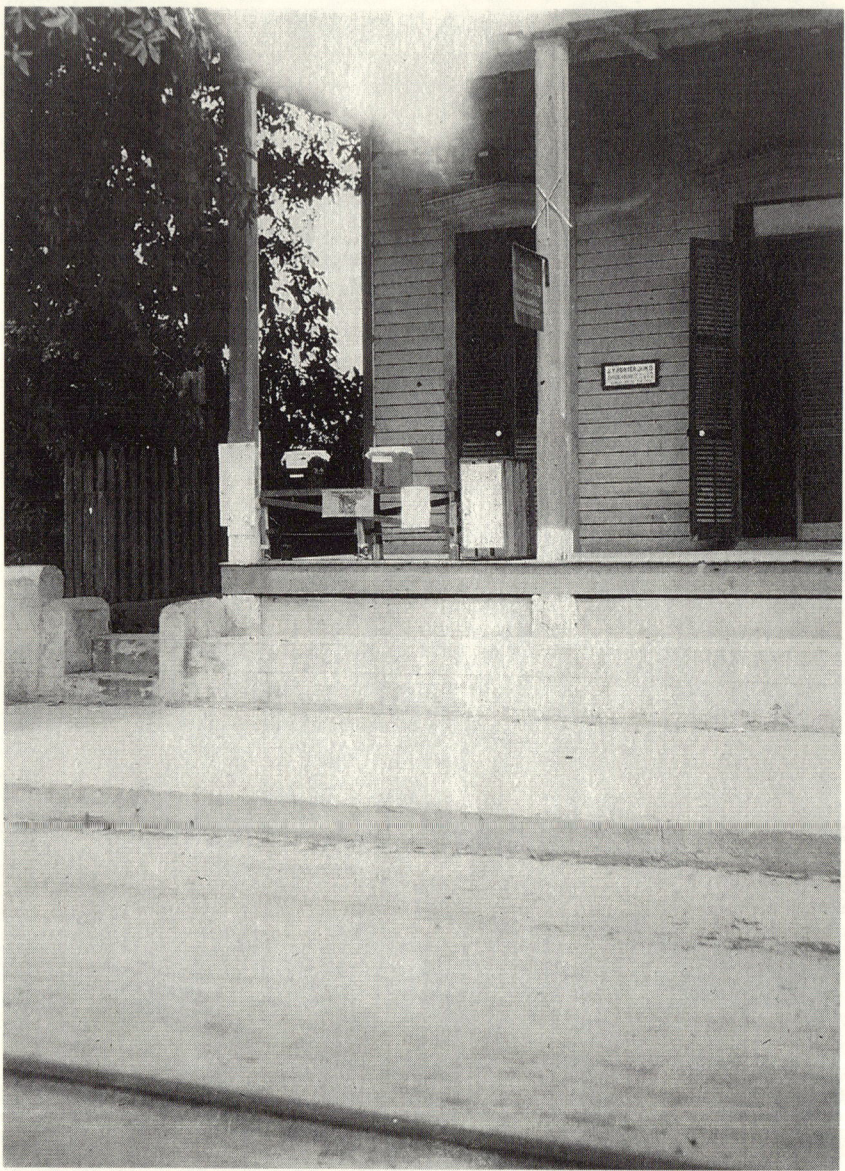

Joseph Y. Porter Jr.'s Fly Exhibit. Source: State Archives of Florida.

The experimentation with the use of exhibition as a pedagogical practice occurred at a critical moment in the history of medicine and society: the rise of the New Public Health. Changes in medical and popular knowledge about disease transmission, changes in immigration and migrations patterns to and within the United States, and changes in the industrial order reshaped public health

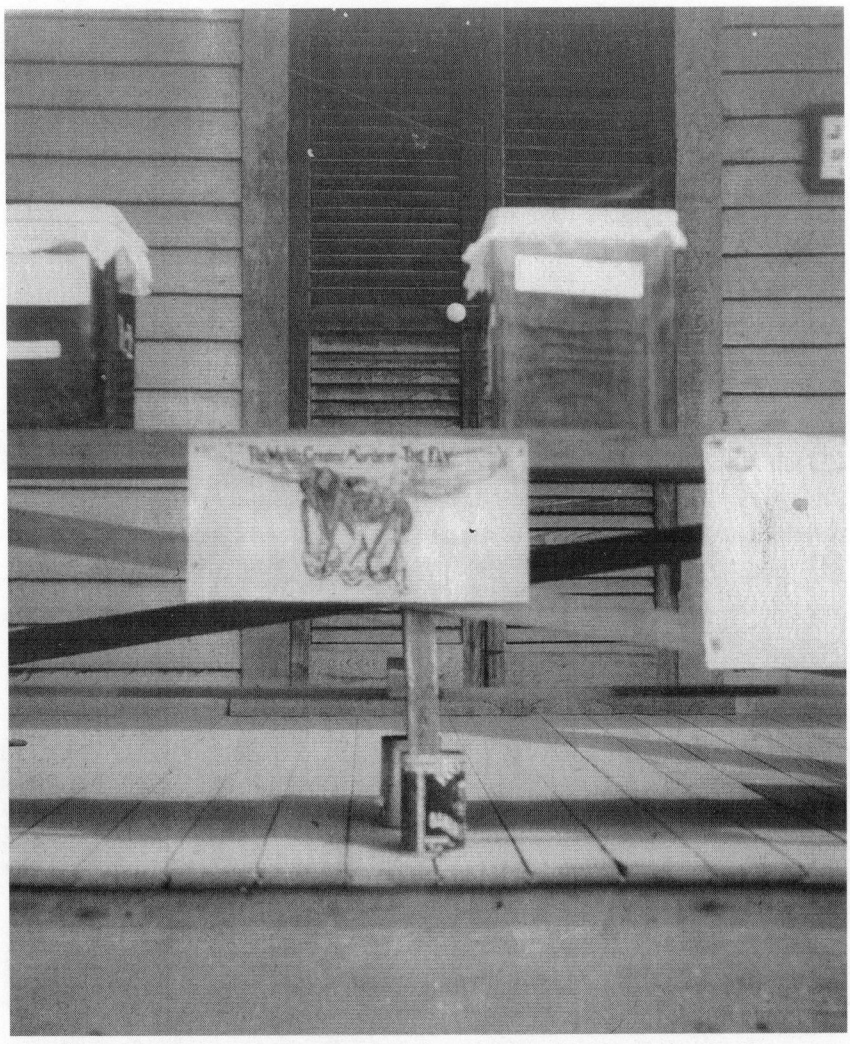

"The World's Greatest Murderer THE FLY." Source: State Archives of Florida.

concerns, notions of who had to be reached, and how. Scientists had identified microbes as the cause of disease. In some cases, this resulted in the creation of cures (syphilis, for instance). In others (tuberculosis, for example), no precise remedy materialized. Instead, prevention at the micro-level appeared to be the most effective way to curtail its spread. Despite the increasing numbers of people living in cities, the late-nineteenth-century strategy of large-scale sanitation projects fell out of favor. Instead, officials turned their focus to convincing people that if they adopted specific individual hygienic behaviors, they could prevent the spread of tuberculosis, yellow fever, hookworm, and other communicable diseases. Gendered expectations and realities led them to market health strategies to women.[4] Statistical studies undergirded health reformers' change in approach. Reports transformed anecdotal evidence about the ill effects of industrialization and urbanization into quantitative proofs. Officials' use of numerical data to demonstrate public health problems extended into rural areas as well. Officials were optimistic that if they could communicate what they knew about scientific specificities, they could create a healthy populace.

However, middle-class reformers' biases toward working-class immigrant men and women (especially those from southern and eastern Europe)—the belief that the majority were stubborn, simple-minded, and unable to process complex textual information—caused them to approach reform with blinders. In doing so, the New Public Health downplayed the systemic structural issues that existed in spaces of poverty that prevented poor people from actualizing disease prevention.[5] Moreover, it rejected any cultural practices deemed at odds with the new orthodoxy. These prejudices also meant that producers of popular health education were inclined to believe that visuals might hold the key to convincing working-class people to change their public health practices voluntarily.

At the turn of the twentieth century, public health officials used many tools to educate the masses: bulletins, illustrated lectures, movies, and temporary exhibits. They viewed mass media in a way similar to many others of the twentieth century, as a "promising tool for democratic ideals."[6] As scholars have noted, these efforts increasingly "privileg[ed] the visual over the textual" to convey medical information.[7] The commodification of anatomical knowledge became a hallmark of professional medical identity and a sign of middle-class status.[8] The circulation of images of the scientist, his laboratory, and medical breakthroughs via mass media positively informed public opinion on the standing of medical professionals and the role of experimental research in fighting disease.[9] Among scientists, film became a research tool.[10] Thus, it was not surprising that health reformers found the idea of using visual representations to communicate public health information alluring.

Exhibiting health was a performative practice in keeping with nineteenth-century dramatizations of the genuine. Nineteenth-century physicians, scientists, and general members of society believed that knowledge could be acquired by studying objects.[11] Personal observation of automaton chess players, FeeJee mermaids, and human oddities led to open discussions about what was "real" and "fake."[12] Trompe l'oeil paintings delivered the illusion of 3-D.[13] In the early twentieth century, world fairs began including displays of "exotic" peoples to elucidate the scientific study of culture.[14] Overall, the use of living bodies lent credence to claims of authenticity.[15] In museums of science, objects had been the foundation of research; now their manner of display mattered.[16]

The reliance on visuals for popular health education converged with the commercialization of popular amusements. World expositions served as essential spaces for combining leisure and health education.[17] Visitors acquired information about changes in theories and practices of medicine by interpreting the various charts, photographs, dioramas, and other sorts of visual displays, which they increasingly expected to be dynamic.[18] In addition to observation, they also learned about modern medicine through the experience of the fair itself.[19]

World fairs and other large exhibitions prompted some reformers to establish permanent institutions for public health research, education, and advocacy. For instance, after seeing the St. Louis World's Exposition, Jane Addams spearheaded the foundation of the Chicago Municipal Museum. The purpose was to make cities livable places for all residents by visualizing strategies for reform.[20] Similarly, a spectacular exhibit on tuberculosis in 1908 spurred the president of the American Museum of Natural History in New York, Henry Fairfield Osborn, to form a Department of Public Health at the museum.[21] Although these experiments in museum making proved influential in shaping public policy, they were short-lived.[22]

Movies also emerged as important spaces to transmit medical beliefs and practices. While urban centers offered the logistical infrastructure and steady stream of consumers to sustain the rise of this new form of popular entertainment, the phenomenon did not stay isolated in cities. Alva Roebuck marketed portable equipment through the Sears, Roebuck catalog, which allowed itinerant entrepreneurs to screen movies in smaller towns across the nation and thereby make a living.[23] Films about public health formed an early mainstay in film catalogs.[24] Martin Pernick has noted, "By the end of the silent film era in 1927, more than 1,300 health-related films had been produced."[25]

Films about tuberculosis, venereal disease, and basic biology were shown in a diversity of spaces ranging from schools to makeshift outdoor venues.[26] The messages remained the same: individual responsibility was the cornerstone of modern disease prevention.[27] Films impressed upon audiences that personal accountability included self-education as much as scruples. In the case with venereal disease films, "'innocent' characters of both sexes g[o]t venereal disease through the lack of scientific knowledge, not just through immorality."[28] As Leslie J. Reagan, Nancy Tomes, and Paula A. Treichler's edited volume, *Medicine's Moving Pictures*, demonstrates, the appeal of using movies as a mechanism for popular education grew throughout the twentieth century.[29]

There were, however, meaningful limits to using film for popular education. The South had fewer movie houses and fewer traveling shows. These constraints stemmed from religious beliefs, infrastructural weaknesses, and Jim Crow restrictions.[30] Also, until the invention of 16-mm film in 1923, the use of movies in formal educational curriculums "remained marginal."[31] My research demonstrates that officials and health reformers more often turned to exhibits than films in their outreach efforts during the first thirty years of the twentieth century. As I will explain in the chapter on health trains, projectors were expensive and cumbersome to move, and in rural areas, there were not enough large-sized electrical public spaces to hold a regular screening. While films projected realism, exhibits allowed audiences to engage directly with tangible things. Movies eventually displaced exhibits but not during the period of this study.

The practices of visual instruction through exhibition that were used for the masses at the world fairs were replicated on a much smaller scale in schools, in lecture halls, and at county and state fairs.[32] Although reformers engaged in national questions about the ills wrought by industrialization, their attempts to respond were local. Consequently, for a time, many social reformers in the early twentieth century engaged in the process of exhibit making.

Reformers borrowed techniques of modern advertising, which combined images and snappy text, to grab the public's attention.[33] They were well aware of "pitchmen['s]" use of similar methods to sell patent medicines.[34] Reformers' success in using new publicity practices to actualize change, however, was hard to measure. Unlike a company, which could calculate the rise and fall of profits in relation to new market strategies, reformers were often at a loss to determine whether awe translated into action. In studying the mid-twentieth century, scholars have concluded that it did not.[35] Moreover, while reformers might have been experts in the study and identification of socioeconomic problems, most were not graphic artists. Learning to create compelling and legible exhibits was not easy.

Providing more information to the public did not necessarily lead to an increase in knowledge.[36] One reason was that over the course of the early twentieth century, medical professionals became less involved with producing materials for popular consumption. Instead, popularization became the purview of journalists.[37] More important, there was a prevailing belief among medical professionals and journalists that the public was incapable of comprehending the erudite aspects of science, and consequently, the goal of "simplification" drove the production of popular educational materials.[38] Using emotion to provoke action became essential to this new form of health instruction.[39]

The impulse to reinvent popular public health education was interrelated to a more general movement to transform educational systems in the

United States. Social reformers hoped that schools would become the nuclei of democracy. They successfully advocated for legislation in many states to make primary education compulsory. They also asserted that schools should serve as spaces to deliver public health services.[40] Social reformers, John Dewey especially, articulated a new approach to the theory of education.[41] Participatory democracy, he argued, rested on participatory education. Students needed to construct meaning for themselves through acts of doing and self-reflection about those experiences. Some museums picked up these new theories of progressive learning.[42] Public health reformers mixed the old and new theories of education into their exhibits. They created spaces to deliver didactic messages and immersive experiences.

Experiential learning was at the heart of another early-twentieth-century innovation for popular health education: the temporary county dispensary. Instituted by the Rockefeller Sanitation Commission (RSC) in its fight against hookworm, the dispensary "resembled an old Southern tent revival" and "revolutionized the way in which the Commission got people to seek treatment."[43] In addition to meeting with a physician, attendees viewed exhibits of images and, in some instances, watched hookworms hatch under microscopes.[44] Although the health exhibit and county dispensary were separate vehicles for instruction, they each contributed to a more general sense that public health education should be participatory.

This study examines the justification and production of exhibits for educating the masses about how to protect the public's health. In the early twentieth century, public health officials and health reformers were optimistic that optical strategies could bring about change. Their use of exhibition occurred at the same time that a new movement in public health emerged, which focused attention away from large-scale projects of environmental infrastructure.[45] Instead, bolstered by the rise of bacteriological knowledge, leaders in public health emphasized the role of individual responsibility in preventing disease transmission. Reformers hoped to teach people the New Public Health using charts, dioramas, and photographs.

Chapter 1 examines the development of the exhibition as a tool for popular education on issues of socioeconomic reform. It uses the most important conduit for communication among reformers across the United States, *Charities and The Commons* (later *The Survey*), to examine the increasing prevalence of exhibits to disseminate information and advocate for change. Tuberculosis exhibits provided the model that other reform groups then followed. Thus, this chapter puts the use of exhibition by public health reformers into context with their peers. It also shows how responses to issues of industrial health, urban planning, and child welfare were infused with public health.

Chapter 2 examines the logic and processes of producing public health displays. It looks at artists who plied their trade making models, the rise of a company that took over the market, and the development of a department at the Russell Sage Foundation that devoted its efforts to disseminating information on best practices for public health exhibits. The individuals and organizations engaged in the art of public health exhibition displayed a deep investment in the aesthetics of these projects. Realism was deemed an essential quality for success. Simplicity was another. Including elements of drama increasingly became seen as advantageous. The goal was to foster engagement without offending anyone's senses or sensibilities. By the 1930s, the standardization of the art of public health exhibition homogenized popular public health education.

Chapter 3 explains how and why public health officials transformed railroad cars into exhibit space through which to distribute consistent medical messages to thousands of people. These health trains crossed the boundaries of urban and rural, wealthy and poor, and, at times, black and white. Health officials and reformers believed that this mode of exhibition served as a mechanism of connectivity to modernity. They also desired them to foster a level of participatory engagement. If only for a brief moment, state officials believed that health trains constituted the most useful tool for popular health education.

Chapter 4 reveals that displaying health sometimes caused a public outcry. Controversial exhibits exposed fault lines between and within communities engaged in public health activities. At times, they also created unlikely alliances. While different content drove the particulars of the various debates about public health displays, the failure of foresight to recognize the existence of significant cleavages between stakeholders remained a standard issue.

In the early twentieth century, public health reformers approached the task of ameliorating unsanitary conditions and preventing epidemic diseases with optimism. Using exhibits, they believed they could make systemic issues visible to masses of people. Embedded within these visual displays were messages about individual action. In some cases, this meant changing hygienic practices. In other situations, this meant taking up action to inform public policy. Reformers and officials hoped that exhibits would energize America's populace to invest in protecting the public's health. This book is an analysis of the logic of production and, where possible, the consumption of this technique for popular health education. It examines the power and limits of using visual displays to support public health initiatives.

Chapter 1

Developing Exhibition as a Common Tool for Popular Education

Residents of East Harlem could window shop for health in 1924. The New York City Department of Health worked with the New York Tuberculosis and Health Association and another "twenty-odd voluntary health and welfare agencies" to create the East Harlem Health Center at 345 East 116th Street. Officials placed rotating exhibits in the Health Shop's storefront to entice the residents of this working-class neighborhood, the majority of whom were Italian, to stop, think, and take action. These visual displays, which sometimes included animatronic models and live demonstrations, provided passersby with information about a myriad of topics ranging from infant care to social hygiene. They also invited residents to step inside for further instruction. The goal was to raise the "consciousness" of the neighborhood to its "health needs" and to formulate positive "health habits."[1]

The Health Shop was an example of how reformers and public health officials began regularly using exhibits as a mechanism to disseminate information about public health with the goal of changing individual hygienic practices and fostering support for governmental apparatuses in the early twentieth century. The target audience for the first aim was working-class immigrants, especially non-English speakers from eastern and southern Europe. The intended audience for the second objective was middle-class men and women, typically white. Reformers viewed their two target groups as interrelated. They believed that responding to infectious diseases, which they statistically associated with urban immigrant neighborhoods, could only be achieved by changing individual health practices, especially in the home. Reformers hoped immigrants would voluntarily adopt new customs such as opening windows at night and brushing

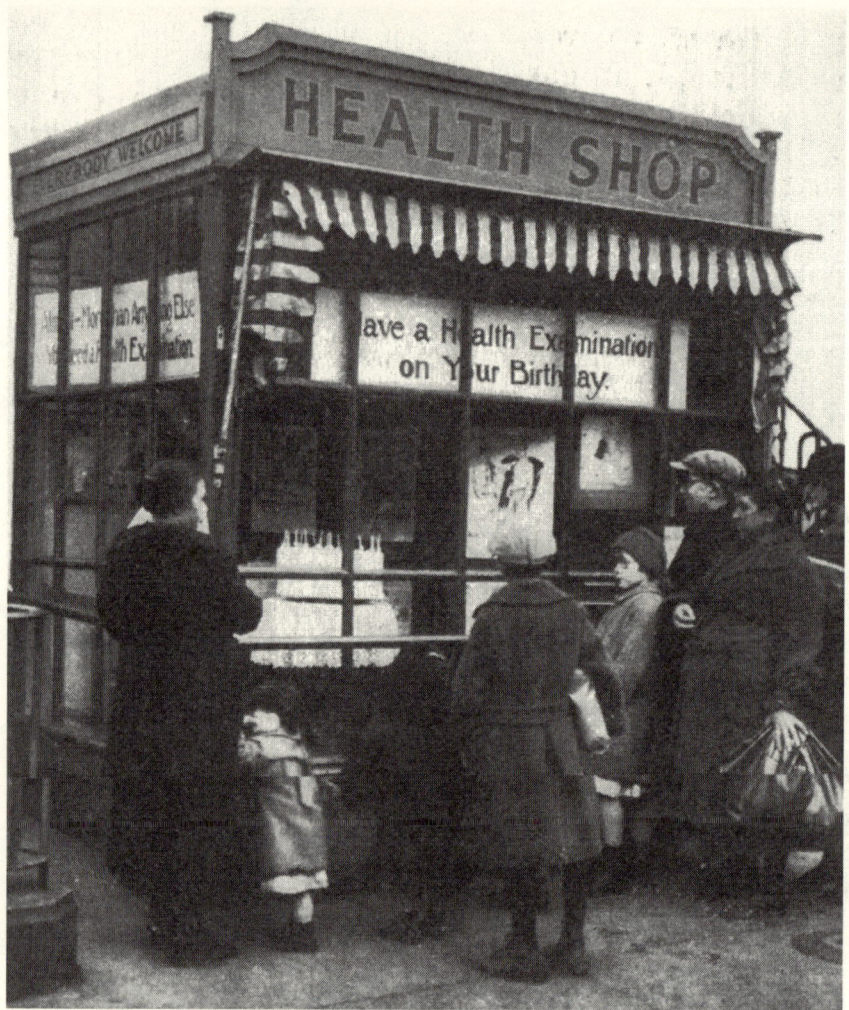

The East Harlem Health Center marketed "health" in its window. Source: *Hygeia* 9,
no. 8 (August 1931).

teeth daily. Reformers' suspicions about immigrants, however, led them to
advocate for the adoption of regulatory controls simultaneously. Spitting on the
street, for instance, became a misdemeanor offense in cities throughout the
nation.

The early twentieth century was a period within which social reformers witnessed remarkable regulatory success. Concerning federal legislation, for
instance, President Theodore Roosevelt signed the Pure Food and Drug Act into
law in 1906. In *Muller v. Oregon*, the U.S. Supreme Court ruled in 1908 that

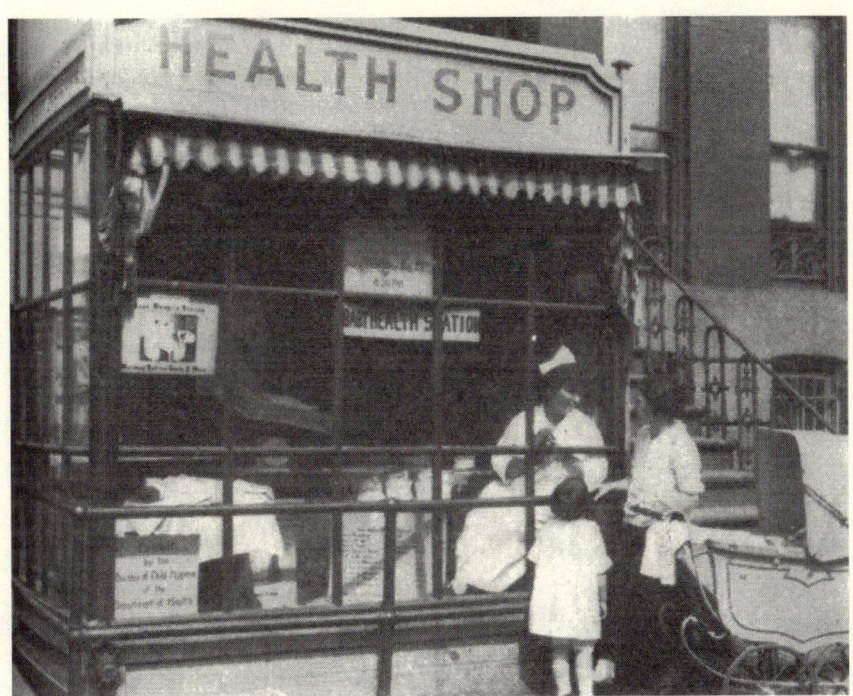

The East Harlem Health Center especially wanted to attract mothers to stop, look, and step inside. Source: *Hygeia* 9, no. 8 (August 1931).

states could limit the number of hours women could work because of the pervading belief that protection of women benefited the public welfare. (Advocates of protective legislation capitalized on the dominant view that regarded women as both a dependent class and as potential mothers of future citizens.[2]) In 1912, Congress established the Children's Bureau. In 1916, Congress passed the Child Labor Law. Successes did not come without setbacks. In 1917, for example, the U.S. Supreme Court found the Child Labor Law to be unconstitutional.

In comparison to changing beliefs about what constituted the rights and responsibilities of citizens through the courts or legislation, exhibits appeared an economical response to the complications of modern capitalism. Many reformers believed that they needed to procure the public's sentiment before they could succeed in securing protective legislation at the state and local levels for addressing health and safety issues related to food and work. Thus, exhibits supported rather than substituted for political action at the state and local levels. At the same time, reformers regarded the persuasive aspects of displays about personal hygiene as a potential failsafe if legislative efforts were reversed.

In general, health reformers and officials believed that visual displays, particularly those that included three-dimensional elements, served as a better mechanism to motivate changes in human behavior then just textual explanations. They thought that sensory materials sculpted sensibilities. Feelings, they assumed, undergirded people's willingness to engage in transformative action. Using exhibits to provide information and act as a means of persuasion, however, was not unique to public health. Many advocates of systemic reform integrated exhibits into their programs for popular education at the beginning of the twentieth century.

An examination of the *Charities and The Commons* (and its successor the *Survey*), which was the communication hub for persons engaged in philanthropic endeavors of a social-service nature, provides documentation of the growing ubiquity of educational exhibitions. Between 1905 and 1928, over one hundred articles appeared in the journal about exhibits the editors believed would be of interest to their readers, who were mostly white and middle class. (There were so many exhibits that in 1913 the *Survey* incorporated a list of them into its classified section.[3]) These accounts described content, outlined goals, and enumerated critiques. Consequently, this periodical provides a critical lens through which to see how reformers conceptualized this new mode of instruction.

This chapter explores the development of the use of exhibition as an ordinary pedagogical tool for progressive reform as documented by the *Charities and The Commons*. It begins with the creation of exhibits on tuberculosis: first, a major exhibit in 1905—the American Tuberculosis Exhibition—and then the smaller exhibits that it inspired. There were several reasons that tuberculosis served as the genesis for this new form of popular education. First, at the turn of the twentieth century, tuberculosis was understood to be the "greatest cause of death" in the United States.[4] Despite a reduction in the mortality rate from tuberculosis by 30 percent by 1920, as many as 10 percent of America's population (15 percent in cities) still succumbed to the disease.[5] Second, the inability of scientists to turn the discovery of the tubercle bacillus into a precise cure meant that physicians relied on relaying proscriptions for prevention to respond to the disease.[6] Approaches to tuberculosis treatment changed throughout the twentieth century as states and sufferers from tuberculosis, armed with new knowledge about the disease, pressed for and against public interventions.[7] Throughout the United States, physicians and laypersons created private organizations to offer advice and services. Municipalities and states also developed systems of surveillance and support for treatment. Private and public concerns often converged. Thus, the advent of exhibits for popular education arrived at the same moment that those looking to prevent the spread of tuberculosis were searching for a mechanism to combine medical information with social persuasion.

Based on the descriptions in the *Charities and The Commons*, it appears that advocates of reform for social-service-related activities used the tuberculosis exhibit as a model to produce exhibits on other social issues. The overlap makes sense in the context of the period. At the turn of the twentieth century, the United States was in the midst of a movement of reform. Middle-class citizens composed a myriad of organizations to bring order to the emerging social and economic circumstances engendered by urbanization and industrialization.[8] Similar to tuberculosis, private organizations took the lead at first and then looked to make partnerships with local and state governments. Although reformers had different ideas about the exact responsibilities of a new activist government (should it be building playgrounds? legislating commerce?), they held a common optimistic belief that they could turn government into a tool for setting standards of living for the benefit of the general welfare.

Judging by the frequency of references in the *Charities and The Commons*, three interest groups in particular introduced exhibition into their reform efforts: urban planning, industrial safety, and child welfare. While different in their specifics, they also often overlapped in the types of materials displayed. Exhibits on urban planning usually included information about antituberculosis campaigns. Exhibits on industrial safety frequently contained data about child labor. Exhibits on child welfare typically incorporated material about tenement reform. Exhibitions, therefore, served as a space of intersection between different foci of reform and often became infused with public health. Reformers shared trust in the ability of exhibits to dramatize dangers and reveal remedies, a faith based on intuition rather than statistical proof, which prompted all of these various groups to invest private and public resources into this mode of popular education.

Tuberculosis as the Template

In late 1905, the National Association for the Study and Prevention of Tuberculosis (NASPT), an organization composed mostly of physicians, and the Committee on Tuberculosis of the New York Charity Organization Society (CSO), an organization comprising primarily laypersons, united to create a major exhibit at the American Museum of Natural History in New York City.[9] It ran from November 27 to December 9 and included materials from around the nation to explain the etiology of tuberculosis, how it spread, how it could be cured, and how individuals could participate in prevention efforts.[10] The goal for the

NASPT was to support the "scientific treatment of tuberculosis."[11] The CSO's mission was to ameliorate a significant cause of poverty.[12] The organizers displayed models, charts, and photographs. They employed docents to explain the contents of the exhibits during the day and held accompanying lectures in the evenings. They also used foreign languages to reach immigrant audiences. The *Charities and The Commons* told its readers that there "can be no manner of doubt of the educational value of" this visual representation of this medical matter.[13] The periodical declared that the impact of examining a "full-sized model of the dark, interior, tuberculosis-breeding bedroom" was more significant than previous strategies (lectures and leaflets) for popular education.[14] Using statistics to measure success, the *Charities and The Commons* noted that the exhibit attracted over 10,000 visitors in the first week it opened.[15]

This exhibit was not the first time education about tuberculosis was put on display, but it was the first exhibit explicitly built to travel.[16] Even before the exhibit closed, reporters noted that the organizers intended to transport it to Boston, Chicago, Newark, and Providence, all cities with large immigrant populations.[17] The exhibit ended up being displayed in whole or in part in large and small cities in the United States as well as traveling to Canada and Mexico.[18] By June 1906, approximately seven months after its initial opening, an estimated 216,000 people had seen the American Tuberculosis Exhibition in some form.[19] In 1907, the Russell Sage Foundation, a philanthropic organization based in New York, provided the resources to "keep the exhibit on the road indefinitely."[20]

Each municipality subtly transformed the exhibit for local interests. In Philadelphia, which displayed the exhibition for two weeks (January 22 to February 3, 1906), organizers placed displays from local institutions purposely toward the entrance. In particular, the pathological exhibits from the Phipps Institute for the Study, Treatment and Prevention of Tuberculosis at the University of Pennsylvania and the Pennsylvania Live Stock Board attracted considerable interest. H.R.M. Landis, a physician affiliated with the Phipps Institute, attributed this to "morbid curiosity."[21] Also, Philadelphians, unlike their New York counterparts, chose to open the exhibit in a vacant downtown department store to entice more foot traffic.

Philadelphia's organizers, however, did not tamper with the overarching message of the exhibit. The goal remained to demonstrate what could be done in everyday situations so that visitors would not "despair because of lack of funds to reach some health resort."[22] Mechanisms for the delivery of information also remained the same. Landis noted that "demonstrators" were present to "explain the special features of the campaign against tuberculosis" and that short lectures were given every evening. Much like New York, Philadelphia's organizers anticipated that not all visitors would be literate in English. In response, at least one address was given in Italian and another in Yiddish.[23] A few months later, Milwaukee adopted a similar strategy. When the American Tuberculosis Exhibition passed through it, "lectures were given in English, German, Polish, and Italian."[24]

In Chicago, which received the exhibit in April 1906, the exhibition was housed in the city's public library in the downtown area. In most respects, the setup in Chicago was similar in content and form to previous installations. For instance, "medical men [were] always in attendance to explain [the pathological display]."[25] Where Chicago differed was in what occurred after the exhibit closed. Instead of packing up the large display and moving on, a smaller traveling exhibit was devised out of the materials to "tour" in the "neighborhood centers in the small parks on the South Side, taking the place of a school garden exhibit."[26]

After Chicago, the idea of taking the tuberculosis exhibit and reformulating it for targeted outreach operations gained popularity. In September 1906, the *Charities and The Commons* noted that the American Tuberculosis Exhibition had spent a week in Manistee, Michigan, which "was a new departure to exhibit in a small town like Manistee."[27] Reportedly, more than 2,000 people (approximately 15 percent of the town's population) came to see the exhibit. The report also noted that some physicians from neighboring towns came to view the materials.[28]

Similarly, in June 1906, the Committee on the Prevention of Tuberculosis of the Charity Organization Society of New York took a truncated version of the exhibit to settlement houses, public halls, and churches throughout the city's boroughs.[29] Placing this new type of storytelling device into intermediary spaces—especially settlement houses—between middle-class reformers and working-class people was important for many reasons. First, organizers believed that every exhibition was an opportunity to cultivate "a group of enlightened and enthusiastic converts from whom permanent help can be expected for the campaign in the future."[30] Second, reformers also hoped that the information in the exhibits would leave each neighborhood with a sense that "tuberculosis and its prevention [was] a matter of common interest which friends and neighbors may talk about together."[31]

Other organizations found this idea appealing. In Minneapolis, the state board of health joined forces with the Minneapolis Associated Charities, Minneapolis Trades and Labor Assembly, the Minneapolis Woman's Club, and the State Federation of Women's Clubs. They created six exhibits to display simultaneously throughout different neighborhoods in the city. They wanted to provide each resident access to the material within walking distance of her and his home.[32]

Community outreach was an essential element in moving to these more intimate locations. Gaylord White, a well-known social worker, explained that New York's organization enlisted the help of "persons of influence" in a neighborhood before opening an exhibit. He denoted these as public school officials, teachers, religious leaders, public health nurses, and physicians. Their goal, White argued, was to sway children between the ages of twelve to fourteen to attend. While White noted that "curiosity" motivated "very young children" to "c[ome] to the door," he explained that exhibitors "excluded" them from participating because the exhibit "could mean little to them."[33] Instead, between peer pressure and the influence of public authority figures, White believed that young adults were more open to actualizing the advice of the exhibit than their younger siblings or their parents.

Although White argued to readers of the *Charities and The Commons* that exhibits were critical educational tools, he also contended that they should not completely replace other methods of communication. He came to this conclusion by eavesdropping. In one instance, he stood looking at a contrast room that showed a space where tuberculosis flourished versus an area where it allegedly would not. Standing next to him were two "young girls" who, "after looking at the "bad" room for a time, inquired seriously, 'what's the matter with it?'"[34] In another instance, White stood in a section with pathological specimens of lungs. Intermixed was a bottle containing cotton that had been placed in a "fresh air flute of a city building."[35] The goal was to demonstrate, in black and white, the poor air quality of the city (i.e., the black one had been exposed to the air). However, White observed "the amateur lecturer, without stopping to read the sign of explanation and casting his eye over the line of lungs, would sometimes pick out this bottle as a horrible example and point to it as a specimen of the frightful pass to which a lung is brought by tuberculosis."[36] White did not trust audiences to interpret the visual displays in the way that their curators intended.

The *Charities and The Commons* concurred with White. The editorial section told readers that although exhibition was an efficient and exciting new mechanism for popular public health education, it should remain a complementary strategy to older ones: "Yet it does not do away with the former methods of educating through lectures and leaflets. These it uses to the fullest extent, but it adds to the printed page and the spoken word, the picture, the photograph, the model."[37] The visual impact of exhibits was significant, but reformers continued to employ traditional didactic methods.

In the years following the initial American Tuberculosis Exhibition, numerous organizations began holding tuberculosis exhibits. The Brooklyn Bureau of Charities, for example, placed a temporary exhibit at Greenpoint Settlement, which served a heavily Polish neighborhood. During its two-week run, an estimated 10,000 people viewed it.[38] In contrast, the Maryland Association for the Prevention and Relief of Tuberculosis desired something more permanent. It created a traveling exhibit that was composed of charts, photographs, pathological specimens, and models. The Association lent the exhibit for one to two weeks to places that had a big enough hall to house it.[39] Sometimes municipalities wanted the benefits of a show but did not want to expend time and money creating their own. Syracuse, for instance, borrowed an exhibit from Boston.[40]

Smaller events did not wholly displace larger ones. Perhaps the grandest exhibit related to tuberculosis occurred in 1908 in Washington, D.C., when the International Congress on Tuberculosis met at the new National Museum. Thirty-three nations sent delegations and six thousand participants registered. In total, 438 organizations contributed exhibits and over a million and a half "sheets of abstracts of papers, printed in Spanish, German, French, and English" were ready for distribution.[41] The *Charities and The Commons* made sure to include numerous images of the various exhibits in its twenty-three-page article about the event.

In describing this exhibit, James F. Lavery, the executive secretary of New York's Tuberculosis Society, told readers that the exhibits showed the work of public and private organizations from around the world.[42] He believed that while exhibits from organizations within the United States had much in common with their global counterparts, Americans emphasized "prevention" in their displays "rather than statistics or cure."[43] He also suggested that Americans stressed the value of the visual in their attempts at popular education.[44] While the exhibit allowed professionals from around the world to share their work, Lavery contended that its "educational value" was greater for the "thousands of popular visitors" who toured the displays.[45]

In 1908, the Board of Aldermen in New York City appropriated funds to secure a redisplay of the international exhibit. The city put up $20,000, and Alfred Meyer, a New York physician with a long history of working on tuberculosis prevention, put up the other $10,000 needed to transport this exhibit from the capital to New York and maintain it for a month.[46] It was a massive exhibit. It required "50,000 square feet of floor space and 100,000 square feet of wall space" and took "more than a thousand packing cases" to transport.[47]

In the subsequent years since the opening of the 1905 exhibit at the American Museum of Natural History (AMNH), reformers found that they had better attendance when they placed exhibits "on a business street or within easy reach of the main lines of city travel."[48] In contrast, the AMNH was located a "distance from the business parts of the city . . . on a quiet" residential street.[49] Consequently, organizers in 1908 initially hoped to house the exhibit in the "new public library at the corner of Fifth Avenue and Forty-second street."[50] However, the library was still under construction, and in the end, they placed the exhibit at the AMNH.

The advertising for the event was immense. Graphic announcements were "plastered" in streetcars, railway cars connecting the suburban area to the city, newspapers, churches, settlement houses, schools, YMCAs, factories, windows of vacant stores, and anywhere else the organizers could get a sign placed.[51] In advertising to potential audiences on the lower East Side of New York, organizers printed cards in Yiddish and English. All of the signs had a double red cross, the symbol of tuberculosis prevention.

The marketing campaign worked. The 1908 tuberculosis exhibit in New York set records for attendance. On its first day, November 30, almost 10,000 people visited the show.[52] By the end of the first week, 145,030 people had walked through its rooms.[53] The final tally of visitors after six weeks was approximately 750,000.[54]

In 1909, E. G. Routzahn, the director of the American Tuberculosis Exhibition of the National Association for the Study and Prevention of Tuberculosis, offered a summary of the past four years of work. According to his records, in 1905, there "were only three exhibits [on tuberculosis] in the entire country."[55] In just a few years, that number had increased exponentially. In 1909, Routzahn counted twenty state-produced exhibits designed for traveling and thirty municipal exhibits. By his accounting, almost three million people had visited one of these various displays.[56] Based on his assessment, the tuberculosis exhibition had become an essential form of popular public health education.

Nonetheless, he cautioned readers of the *Survey* that exhibition was "in no sense a revolutionary force."[57] Unlike other tools of progressive reform that used mathematical proofs to demonstrate problems and offer solutions, Routzahn argued that exhibits "cannot bring 'results' to be tabulated and exploited."[58] Instead, he believed that tuberculosis exhibitions were "expected to awaken interest, to impart information, to lead to activity, and to suggest work to be done and plans for doing it."[59] The goal, he contended, was "to stimulate" work in both antituberculosis and other health-related reform activities.[60] Looking at the use of exhibits related to urban planning, industrial safety, and child welfare suggests that Routzahn's hope was at least partially fulfilled.

Vol. XXI. No. 16   January 16, 1909

CHARITIES
AND The Commons

A WEEKLY JOURNAL OF PHILANTHROPY AND SOCIAL ADVANCE

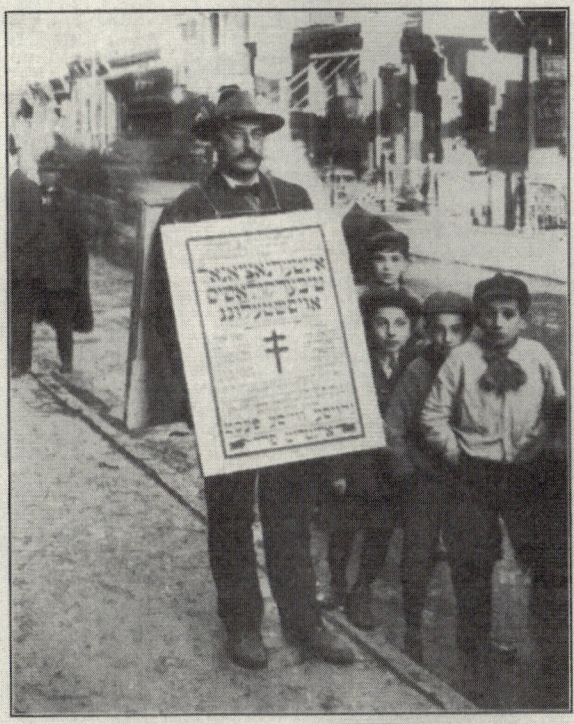

ADVERTISING THE TUBERCULOSIS EXHIBIT ON NEW YORK'S EAST SIDE
The sandwich-man, furnished by the Bureau for the Handicapped, has only one arm

Charity Organization Society of the City of New York
Robert W. deForest, President; Otto T. Bannard, Vice-President; J. P. Morgan, Treasurer; Edward T. Devine, General Secretary

105 East 22d Street   174 Adams Street
New York   Chicago

ENTERED AT THE POST OFFICE
NEW YORK, N. Y. AS
SECOND-CLASS
MATTER

This Issue Ten Cents a Copy   Two Dollars a Year

Organizers needed to advertise exhibits in multiple languages if they wanted to attract a diverse audience. In this case, the sign is printed in Hebrew to attract Jewish residents of New York's Lower East Side of Manhattan. Source: *Charities and The Commons* 21, no. 16 (January 16, 1909).

Urban Planning

Social reformers of the late nineteenth and early twentieth centuries were interested in how they could apply scientific study to what they believed were the negative consequences of urban living: substandard housing, inconsistent garbage collection, air pollution, and a compromised food supply. Female reformers, in particular, were concerned with the creation and management of infrastructure to make cities livable.[61] Reformers used exhibits to make compelling arguments about how to recognize and address urban ills. Cities used exhibits to justify public expenditures.

The first mention in the *Charities and The Commons* of an exhibit related explicitly to urban planning was in 1905. Inspired by the Model Street exhibits at the world's fair in St. Louis in 1904, reformers in Chicago desired a space "devoted to the collection and interpretation of material illustrating the physical and social conditions and the administration of cities."[62] With the renowned reformer Jane Addams spearheading the project, Chicago's reformers created a Municipal Museum in February 1905 and found housing in Chicago's Public Library.[63] The museum presented material on numerous issues related to the management of cities: clean water, sewage, food supply, street cleaning, smoke abatement, garbage collection, and public transportation. These were all temporary exhibits on loan from various organizations, including for several weeks the American Tuberculosis Exhibition. Lenora Austin Hamlin, an experienced curator who directed the museum, hoped that space would become a "dynamic university" that would "teach its lessons through the eye rather than through the ear and the printed page; selecting, valuing and placing the emphasis by the use of color and form."[64] Despite assertions of success, after a year, the library reclaimed the space for its other needs.[65]

The next reference to an exhibit focused on urban planning in the *Charities and The Commons* appeared three years later. In 1908, New York witnessed "the Exhibit of Congestion of Population," which the American Museum of Natural History housed for two weeks in March. The organizers displayed information about what they believed to be the causes and adverse effects of congestion within the city.[66] In particular, the exhibit included information about tuberculosis, crime, and substandard housing. The exhibition contended that all of these problems stemmed from overcrowding. It attempted to support that argument with maps, diagrams, charts, statistics, models, and photographs. Upon touring the exhibit, the governor of New York, Charles Evans Hughes, remarked that he felt both "oppressed and depressed by the facts" presented in the exhibit on the "wretchedness and misery which are incident to our progress."[67] The exhibit argued that the present piecemeal approach of charity (churches and settlements) was insufficient.[68] Instead, organizers contended that only municipalities could coordinate the systemic change based on scientific methods necessary for permanent amelioration.

The following year, New York witnessed another exhibit related to urban ills when the City Planning Exhibition opened at the Twenty-second Regiment Armory at 1988 Broadway Avenue in May 1909. Two associations organized it. The Committee on Congestion of Population, which had been formed in 1908 by over a hundred people from different groups, engaged in some activity related to antipoverty programs in New York City, and the Municipal Art Society, took a leading role in preaching the benefits of the City Beautiful movement.[69] Charles Mulford Robinson, a famed urban theorist, reviewed the exhibit in the *Survey*. Although his overall impression was positive, he levied some sharp criticisms against the overall format. For instance, Robinson looked for an overarching narrative but did not find one. This left him unsure how to navigate the exhibit space. He told his audience that the "entrance to the hall was not inviting, and if one were so lucky as to begin his study of the exhibits at the right place, the opening impression was not propitious."[70]

In addition to issues of steering, Robinson warned potential curators about the problems of messaging. If this exhibit's goal was to encourage faith in the social capacity of government, he believed that its structure might have done the opposite. Robinson described the incongruity. A visitor encountered an aisle with two cards at its entrance. The sign on one side said, "Taxation is Democracy's Most Effective Method of Securing Social Justice." The opposite side said, "If the City Secured by Taxation a Large Part of the Increase in Land Values, Congestion would Lose Most of its Charm." Robinson argued that these two cards "immediately put the average man on defensive" because he might believe that he was "getting into something socialistic, and, quite possibly having some interest in land and certainly in taxes, was on his guard."[71]

Nevertheless, Robinson believed that in its entirety, the exhibition articulated a convincing argument about the benefits of urban planning, especially concerning public health. One aisle, for instance, was devoted entirely to a display from the Brooklyn Committee on Prevention of Tuberculosis. Also on display were the results of the Pittsburgh Survey, with which readers of the *Charities and The Commons* would have been familiar.[72] The exhibit presented the efforts of Berlin and Glasgow to plan transportation routes, restrict industrial sites from residential ones, and develop public spaces for leisure activities.[73] Lastly, Honolulu, Boston, and other cities from around the nation exhibited their efforts to cope with urban growth.[74]

As municipalities increasingly took on new roles, it seemed pertinent to explain how cities spent tax dollars.[75] In 1910, the *Survey* noted that cities began holding "Budget" Exhibitions. The goal was to "acquaint" people on the "manner in which public business [was] conducted."[76] The *Survey* reported on exhibits in New York, Toledo, Hoboken, and Cincinnati. Each had displays related to various aspects of public service, typically fire, police, and street sanitation.[77] Still, there were aspects presented that were unique to each municipality. Hoboken, for instance, included a relief map to demonstrate how high tide flooded parts, making a gravity-sewage system impractical.[78]

In 1911, New York City attempted to innovate this topic by integrating short films into its displays. The city believed this would be a dynamic way to explain to its residents how the city spent almost two hundred million dollars each year. Although it did not state who made the movies or how they were created, (staged or candids) visitors could watch "The Docking of the Olympic, How the Police Dogs Capture Runaway Criminals, Police Riot Drill, and How the Police Care for a Lost Child."[79] The combination presented civic dollars in action.

In describing a similar exhibit in Milwaukee, readers of the *Survey* were told that its purpose was "to satisfy the curiosity of citizens to know just what the city gives them in exchange for the taxes they pay."[80] Displays included information about tuberculosis, child welfare, regulation of food supplies, building inspection, the public library, museum, and the department of public works. According to the review in the *Survey*, the exhibit was both "spectacular and scientific."[81]

Sometimes cities held exhibits about one particular issue of urban living. Pittsburgh, for instance, held a smoke abatement exhibit in 1913. Organized by the Smoke Abatement League of Pittsburgh, the exhibition attempted to demonstrate the social and economic costs of this type of pollution. One representation was of side-by-side obelisks, one of the Washington Monument and next to it a darker, significantly taller, twin monument depicting the volume of soot that fell on Pittsburgh in 1912.[82]

While not as numerous as tuberculosis exhibits, displays of urban planning served a similar purpose. City officials and reformers attempted to communicate information by combining texts, photographs, charts, and models. One goal was to make issues of urban living that proved detrimental to the health and welfare of residents visible. A second aim was to present arguments about the capabilities of citizens and municipalities to intervene.

Industrial Safety

Advocates of industrial-safety reform drew direct inspiration from the American Tuberculosis Exhibition. Writing to its readers in 1906, the *Charities and*

The Commons declared that upon seeing the "work undertaken by the travel-ing exhibit of the National Tuberculosis Association . . . it [was] difficult to see how public sentiment could be more effectively molded to work for the aboli-tion of the sweatshop and child labor, north and south, than by holding indus-trial exhibitions."[83] Where industrial-safety exhibits came to differ from tuberculosis and urban planning exhibits was in their growing use of live demonstrations.

The first reference in the *Charities and The Commons* related to an exhi-bition on industrial safety appeared in July 1906 when the American Institute of Social Service (AISS) announced its intention to hold an event at the Ameri-can Museum of Natural History on "safety devices and industrial hygiene."[84] The AISS was founded in 1902 in New York by those who, in response to "the modern industrial revolution," wished to form an organization to put "human experience on file" and "make it available to all who desire to profit by the expe-rience of others."[85] AISS wanted to present manufacturers with full-sized mod-els of the latest technological advances in safety equipment. Four "museums of security" already existed for such purpose in Europe, one in Amsterdam, Munich, Berlin, and Paris.[86] AISS hoped that seeing how devices worked would con-vince manufacturers that the expense was worth the investment.

AISS especially wanted to display automatic cutoff devices. AISS believed their installation was critical because of the multilingual demographics of Amer-ica's workforce. They cited an example of a recent lethal accident in a steel factory as evidence. AISS argued that a "rapidly moving bar of iron at white heat . . . r[a]n through [the] body" of an Italian worker for two reasons. First, he did not understand the "shouts of his fellow workers." Second, he also could not "read the conspicuously placed warnings" because they were in English.[87]

AISS hoped that this temporary exhibit could be crafted into a permanent American Museum of Security. AISS believed that the institution could serve as a collection point for information related to industrial safety. This informa-tion could then be used to influence public policy: "It would lay before state legislatures the importance of requiring a strict report of all accidents."[88]

Industrial exhibits used models, photographs, charts, and graphs in ways similar to that of tuberculosis exhibits and urban planning exhibits. They often also used docents. For instance, although every presentation at the Philadelphia Industrial Exhibition was "placarded" in a manner which "spoke clearly for themselves," organizers also used a "group of young women" to act as "guides" in providing explanations.[89] Industrial exhibits also increasingly used full-size dioramas complete with living displays to dramatize haphazard working conditions.

In reviewing the Philadelphia Industrial Exhibition for the *Charities and The Commons*, theater expert Mabel Hay Barrows Mussey noted that the exhibits that drew the greatest crowds were the ones with real-time presentations. She described three different "fac-simile" rooms. In the first, an Italian woman sat stripping carpet rags accompanied by her six-year-old son and baby. According to Mussey, "here all the usual conditions had been faithfully retained, even to the little boy's dirty face."[90] In another room, the Central Labor Union displayed a sweatshop in action. Next to the sweatshop was a room with two women, "finishers," with a baby in between them. Mussey was struck by the "essence of realism" in the display "even with the breadknife lying on the bed, within reach of the baby."[91] These displays, she argued, made visible what reformers contended were dangers hidden from the public's view.

The goal, Mussey claimed, was to make middle-class consumers feel responsible for the conditions of production. One placard, for instance, stated that "this suit is being made for a fashionable tailor—it may be yours."[92] In case anyone doubted the veracity of the depictions, the *Charities and The Commons* assured readers that the "facts used in all cases have been taken from photographs and on each booth will be displayed the photograph from which the exhibit was prepared."[93] Mussey used her authority as a theatrical expert to dismiss questions about the scripted nature of this reality show. Editorial manipulation of photographs to advance particular arguments was not exceptional. On several occasions, the *Survey* captioned Lewis Hine's photographs with its own interpretation of what the editors believed was significant about the image.[94]

Organizers of industrial-safety exhibits, much like their counterparts, defined success based on attendance numbers and hoped that exhibits would engender public policy initiatives. For instance, the *Charities and The Commons* told readers that despite an admission fee of a quarter (approximately 5 dollars in today's relative value), attendance at the Chicago Industrial Exhibit "increased from day to day," and it was so high the last few evenings that it "taxed the capacity" of the venue.[95] At the mass meeting on the last day, those in attendance adopted resolutions calling for the state legislature to enact legislation that offered workers greater protection.

Similar to the tuberculosis model, organizers of industrial-safety exhibits often shared materials. Chicago, for example, recycled materials from the Philadelphia exhibit. Organizers also secured materials from New York's "exhibit of protected machinery and safety devices in industry."[96] In this way, what was sometimes a local story became a national one.

In promoting the Chicago Industrial Exhibit, organizers connected issues of worker safety with consumers' concerns. One advertisement that appeared in street cars asked riders to consider whether they would allow people with consumption or scarlet fever to cook their meals or make their clothes in their homes: "Have you a consumptive cook? Or has your seamstress the scarlet fever? Not in your kitchen, of course, or in your sewing room but do you know about the basement bakeries and sweatshops where your bread and clothes may come from?" To learn how to distinguish the "good and the bad," the placard argued, attend the Industrial Exhibit at Brooke's Casino.[97]

Similar to Philadelphia, Chicago also created rooms with living tableaus of substandard workspaces. They built a house with open windows, with each room containing a different issue. One had an Italian mother and her four children shelling nuts for $3.00 a week. Next door was an Italian man and woman finishing garments in their "home."[98] The *Charities and The Commons* devoted an entire page to a photograph of the life-sized and life-staffed display. The journal, however, did not report on the controversy that ensued over this exhibition. Some of the participants objected to the negative way in which they were being displayed and refused to continue performing.[99]

Graham Taylor, the founder of the settlement the Chicago Commons, wrote about the experience of being at the exhibit. In particular, he made notes about the audience. Of the 10,000 who visited the exhibition, he believed that approximately two-thirds were trade unionists, whom he characterized as "plain folk."[100] He arrived at this conclusion because trade unions had actively participated in creating the exhibits and promoted them to workers. Taylor viewed the exhibition as a place to foster mutual understanding between producers and consumers: "People were made to realize the extent to which the interests and welfare of wage earners are co-incident with the interests and welfare of the whole people. And conversely the trade unionists learned the value of a closer acquaintance with public sentiment—learned its desire to know the facts and be fair."[101] Taylor argued that exhibit halls served as public squares.

His experience was borne out in Massachusetts, where the state borrowed materials from the American Institute on Social Service to hold an Industrial Exhibit in Boston in April 1907.[102] Writing about the exhibit, Edward T. Hartman of the Massachusetts Civic League noted that not all visitors to the exhibition needed displays to learn about dangerous conditions. In showing a safety device for a planer, the docent who was explaining its value told Hartman that "no less than thirty men, after looking at the machine, held up mutilated fingers and hands and remarked, 'this I got through lack of that.'"[103] Hartman, nevertheless, worried that visitors might not be able to decipher the messages of the exhibit. He contended that there were too many details: "Diagrams, charts and statistics there were in abundance, but their significance was lost on many."[104]

The National Child Labor Committee (NCLC), which was founded in 1904 by reformers from around the nation concerned about the mental, physical, and emotional well-being of children, created presentations that often contained visuals that combined information about industrial safety, urban planning, child welfare, and public health.[105] Readers of the *Survey* would have been informed about those connections if they had read the article about NCLC's exhibit on "Home Work" that it presented at the Women's Industrial Exhibition in New York in March 1912. This particular display gave graphs, charts, and photographs of a study by the New York State Factory Investigating Committee, which examined the "immunity" of tenements from legislation related to workers' safety and child labor.[106] The survey of tenements at night, 1,037 visits to be precise, documented how children worked into the evening performing labor. A Lewis Hine photograph, for instance, captured children making dolls to be sold at Christmas.[107] Additional images purported to demonstrate a direct relationship between home work and the spread of infectious diseases: "Several showed a tubercular woman at work, a tubercular boy in the room with home workers, and other families of workers in which children were sick with mumps and measles."[108] This exhibit made clear that there was considerable overlap between public health and industrial safety.

Child Welfare

Child welfare exhibits followed similar patterns as urban planning and industrial safety. Organizers used photographs, charts, models, and docents to make their case that children's issues were a public matter. These exhibits were also very interdisciplinary. Child welfare exhibits often included public health information, especially on tuberculosis, material on child labor, and questions about the quality of living quarters. This type of display was also particularly popular in the two years leading up to the creation of the federal Children's Bureau in 1912. The organizers of these events were usually women, which paralleled the broader movement by women to develop civic infrastructure to protect the health and welfare of women and children.[109]

In 1910, the *Survey* began reporting on the preparations for a large child welfare exhibit to take place in early 1911 in New York City. The goal, according to the journal, was to be "more vivid and dramatic than others given of late years."[110] While the *Survey* did not provide many details about this particular exhibit, the journal did extensively report on its aftermath. In particular, the *Survey* described the ways that the display traveled.

After seeing the exhibit in New York, Nancy McCormick, wife of Cyrus H. McCormick, who made his fortune on having invented a mechanical reaper, decided to bring the exhibit to Chicago by financing its transport and display with a gift of $50,000.[111] In this way, she was doing what many other peers were doing, especially in Chicago.[112] She used her elitism to support progressive reform causes related to women and children. However, she wanted to do more than bring the current exhibition. She wanted to expand it. Chicago's version of the Child Welfare Exhibit was to be the most substantial cooperative creation in the city since the Columbian Exposition.[113] The exhibit was installed at the Coliseum, which, at 72,000 square feet, was double the space New York's version had used when it occupied the Seventh Regiment Armory.[114] Chicago employed 1,500 "explainers" to act as "guides" to attendees.[115] In the two weeks that it was open, organizers counted 420,000 visitors.[116]

Chicago writer I. K. Friedman recorded impressions, his own and those around him, which the *Survey* then printed. Overall, Friedman believed that the exhibition presented "scientific talks in simple language" and that it gave the information through "objects rather than words."[117] He described looking at materials related to homes, playgrounds, museums, libraries, schools, and public health. He wrote about a "living exhibit" composed of the industrial arts and domestic science being taught to fifth- and sixth-grade boys and girls. The girls cooked and sewed. The boys did carpentry, pottery, bookbinding, printing, weaving, and basketry.[118] Friedman described some models in Chicago's Department of Health exhibit. For instance, the department displayed 3,500 dolls to illustrate the 3,500 annual deaths of children in the city. Next to this static display was a more dynamic one related to infant mortality. A line of figures, four to a row, marched forward. At a certain moment, the fourth figure "was cut down and removed from sight" to illustrate that "only three in every four infants 'grew up.'"[119]

Anita McCormick Blaine, daughter of Nancy and Cyrus McCormick and an activist in progressive causes, gave the keynote address. In it, she acknowledged the work of philanthropists whose contributions were on exhibit. She "conced[ed] the essential value" of the child welfare work "carried on by private philanthropy."[120] Nonetheless, she argued that building an infrastructure to promote and protect children's welfare rightly belonged as a civic function. The *Survey* summarized her position: "she placed supreme emphasis upon the city as the only agency which is both obligated and equipped to meet the common needs for all its children."[121]

After Chicago, other cities booked the Child Welfare Exhibit, including Montreal, which was set to open the exhibit in October 1912. In reporting on this event, organizers believed that the city's rapid growth—which they estimated at 25,000 to 40,000 annually—had resulted in issues of congestion. They calculated an astronomical rate of childhood mortality; "of the children born in Montreal, 54.92 per cent die before reaching the age of five."[122] Organizers hoped that audiences in Montreal would be as stimulated as those in Chicago and New York to take action to change conditions in their city.

The exhibit also inspired other cities to begin holding their own child welfare shows. Kansas City, for instance, staged an exhibition in December 1911. Given under "municipal auspices," Kanas City's Board of Public Welfare organized the exhibit.[123] The five-member all-male board had been organized in 1910 to "fulfill the duties of the City toward all the poor, the delinquent, the unemployed, the deserted and the unfortunate classes in the community and to supervise the private agencies which solicited money from the public for these purposes."[124] William Volker, the former head of the board and a well-known businessman who made his fortune in home furnishings, funded the exhibit.[125] The *Survey* noted that in some respects, the materials presented were similar to those seen in Chicago and New York. However, the anonymous reviewer of the exhibit believed that in three ways, Kansas City's presentation was different. First, the correspondent felt that Kansas City wanted every single visitor to experience a "prick" to force them to acknowledge the negative issues of life within their community.[126] Second, the reporter asserted that the exhibit was imbued with "western optimism," although he or she did not specify what that meant.[127] Third, the writer noted that the exhibit "did not adhere quite so strictly to the subject of child welfare" like New York and Chicago. For instance, it included materials related to factory work for young women, especially the problem of meager wages.

Big exhibits inspired smaller exhibits. In Chicago, similar to the creation of a traveling display on tuberculosis, the Woman's City Club put together a smaller version of the child welfare exhibit to make available for "neighborhood display in all parts of Chicago."[128] In particular, they hoped that these "civic exhibits" would be brought to "schools, small park recreation centers, and other common meeting places of the people."[129]

In 1913, May Ayres, who worked in the Division of Education for the Russell Sage Foundation, reported on Rochester's experience because afterward, organizers (she did not specify as to who exactly they were) did something different from their predecessors.[130] Organizers conducted a visitor's survey of their Child Welfare Exhibit and shared their analysis of the results with Ayres, who then shared them with readers of the *Survey* (and newspapers across the country republished the results).[131] They hoped that this would allow other organizers to determine effective messaging to their target audience, young adults.

Rochester's organizers asked students "in the upper grades" to write letters about what they remembered seeing at the exhibit. They collected 553 letters and analyzed their contents. Where evidence suggested that teachers had edited the letters, the organizers discarded them. Within the letters, organizers looked for references to different exhibit features. Based on the notes, the "most impressive single exhibit seems to have been that of the tidy and untidy home."[132] The contrast of the "clean and dirty markets" also garnered a significant number of comments probably because of its vivid depiction of blood dripping from a cow's head. "Helen" described the scene in her letter as thus: "In the good store the store keeper was dressed in white, the food all looked clean and in a nice glass case. In the bad store the cat was on the counter and the celery and lettuce was all dried up, and the rest is too disgusting to tell about."[133]

In reviewing the letters for positive and negative feedback, the organizers found the overwhelming majority to be favorable. They did, however, see that some children found the conditions of the exhibit experience unfavorable. A number found the space too overcrowded and stuffy as a result.[134] Most of the letters reprinted in the *Survey* were descriptive of what they saw. A few, though, remarked that they were taking different actions at home based on what they had seen. For instance, "Maurice" stopped drinking coffee based on the exhibits. An unnamed eleven-year-old girl wrote that she would put the information about baby care to use on vacation because it was going to be her job to "take care of the baby."[135] Lastly, one child concluded what organizers believed "many other observers ha[d] reached before her: 'The impression of the whole exhibit on me was that it is slow work.'"[136]

Within just a few years of the first exhibit opening, the *Survey* remarked, "local child welfare exhibits are becoming so numerous that the movement has attained national scope."[137] In response, the National Child Welfare (NCW) Exhibition Committee, which was headquartered in New York, offered to work with local communities to lend them materials. The NCW's exhibit was built to travel. It was fifteen feet in length and divided into seven sections: "material on sex education and hygiene; the school building; vocational education; homemaking and assimilation; the dependent child; the child's food; public recreation and social centers."[138] It could be lent in whole or in part. At the time of the article, the exhibit was on loan to the Children's Bureau, where it was displayed in the context of a National Conservation Exhibit.

Conclusion

In the early twentieth century, reformers interested in social-service-related activities began to use exhibition with greater frequency to deliver popular education. The *Charities and The Commons* provided readers across the nation with a sense of the diversity of these exhibits, the utility of presentations for communicating messages, and, in few cases, the limits of the exhibition. The journal documented exhibits ranging from modest displays to spectacular spectacles.

Public health was central to the development of the use of exhibition as a tool for popular education. Tuberculosis exhibits set the model. Models, photographs, and charts were essential features. Increasingly, exhibits contained living objects. In case seeing did not result in believing, reformers engaged docents to interpret the scientific aspects of displays. Reformers believed that the emotive elements of presentation would prompt action. In the case of middle-class men and women, reformers hoped visitors would walk away with a desire to support an expansion of government regulation and apparatuses to respond to quality-of-life issues. In the case of working-class immigrants new to the United States, reformers hoped the visual displays would prompt visitors to change individual hygienic behaviors in the home, work, and public spaces.

The *Charities and The Commons* tells a story of creation and dissemination but not of production and consumption. The chapters that follow analyze the artistry of exhibition, the elaboration of exhibition, and the contested nature of exhibition. The use of this visual mechanism for popular public health education was in step with other reform movements but, as will become clear, also came with its own particularities.

Chapter 2

The Art of Exhibit Making

In 1915, Joseph Y. Porter, Florida's chief health officer, wrote to Willard Knowlton, director of the New Jersey Board of Health, to inquire about New Jersey's use of models to communicate information to the public about diets for consumptives.[1] In response, Knowlton sent two prints of a food exhibit he had created as a table-top display and provided information on the artist, Julius Heinrich of Baldwin, Long Island. Heinrich worked as a model maker for the Peter Henderson Seed Company, which was where Knowlton "discovered him."[2] Knowlton believed that new models could be made from existing molds. Porter thanked Knowlton for the information but decided that the models were too large for his purposes. Still, Porter was hopeful that Heinrich could modify them for Florida.[3]

Knowlton and Porter's ad hoc approach to exhibit production was typical of this historical period. In seeking artistry related to public health issues, health officials cast their nets wide. As a result, artists from a range of disciplines and commercial ventures, as demonstrated by Heinrich, found demand for their services. Health officials and reformers believed they had identified a mechanism with which to connect their goals to an emerging consumer culture, especially using three-dimensional objects that gave the appearance of being alive. At the same time, they needed to contend with art as a business. Thus, the art of exhibit making was a process of trial and error for artists, officials, and health reformers.

In the early twentieth century, exhibition became a favorite medium through which to convey public health knowledge. Reformers and government officials used visual displays to promote the positive impact of public policy on health.[4]

Contemporaries noted the opportunities this provided for the "scientific arti-san."[5] While a commercial market for medical wares already existed, public health exhibition opened up a new space for physicians to display their depictions of anatomy, and companies found a new sales floor for medical models.[6]

For a time, making models for public health demonstrations was a lucrative business. In addition to representing the human body, artisans were called upon to create drawings and models of sanitation structures, the process of disease transmission, and depictions of personal hygienic practices. Still, there were only a few specialists engaged in the trade. In 1914, Evart G. Routzahn, associate director of the Russell Sage Foundation's Department of Surveys and Exhibits (which was created in 1912 and is discussed later in this chapter), counted eleven model makers who specialized in public health display, eight of whom worked in New York City.[7] (Heinrich was not on the list.) After further research, Routzahn added two more, both of whom worked in Washington, D.C.[8]

This chapter examines the logic and processes of producing medical models for public health displays. It looks at two artists who plied their trade making models, the rise of a company that took over the market, and the development of a department at the Russell Sage Foundation led by Routzahn that devoted its efforts to disseminating information on best practices for public health exhibits. The individuals and organizations engaged in the art of public health exhibition displayed a deep investment in the aesthetics of these projects. Realism was deemed an essential quality for success. Simplicity was another. Including elements of drama increasingly became seen as advantageous. If a living object could not be produced, mimicry was desired. The goal was to foster engagement without offending anyone's senses or sensibilities.[9] By the 1930s, the standardization of the art of public health exhibition homogenized popular public health education.

Scientific Artisans: Philipp Rauer and Mica Heidemann

This section focuses on two model makers, Philipp Rauer and Mica Heidemann (Rauer was on Routzahn's list, Heidemann was not). Their stories illustrate the methodological, ethical, and financial issues involved in crafting artifakes for display. Each marketed his or her wares on the lifelike nature of his or her representation. Each found himself or herself very busy for a brief period. Lastly, each made a significant amount of money from his or her models. However, the highly customized and expensive nature of their art put their vocation at risk once a company began mass-producing materials. Lastly, their tales demonstrate the contingent character of this work.

In 1914, the Rockefeller Sanitation Commission for the Eradication of Hookworm Disease (RSC) ceased operating in the U.S. South, as international efforts became a new priority.[10] The end of operations did not mean, however, that the Rockefeller Foundation desired to relegate the RSC's domestic work to the dustbin of history. Instead, the International Health Commission (IHC), successor to the RSC, decided to showcase the RSC's work at the Panama-Pacific International Exposition to be held in San Francisco in 1915. This event was the IHC's first foray into creating a major exhibit, and its administrators hired Philipp Rauer, an Austrian physician working in Germany who was known for making spectacular medical models, to ensure success.

Despite the existence of American specialists, the general perception in the United States was that Europeans possessed a vastly greater skill set.[11] In the 1930s, Germans, in particular, were viewed as experts in "visualizing health."[12] Their techniques offered an aseptic interaction between viewer and object, which made their exhibits suitable for intermixes of men, women, and children.[13] Despite the failure of these exhibits to fundamentally change people's public health behaviors, they were awe-inspiring.[14]

Philipp Rauer secured fame as an artisan of public health displays for his work on "Der Mensch," an exhibit on the internal workings of the human body at the International Hygiene Exhibit in Dresden in 1911.[15] King Leopold of Belgium and Emperor William II of Germany awarded honors to Rauer for his fabrications. This recognition led him to the attention of Alvin E. Pope, the head of the Departments of Education and Social Economy for the Panama-Pacific International Exposition that was to be held in San Francisco in 1915. Pope wrote to Wickliffe Rose, head of the IHC, that Pope "would be able to secure enough work to keep Herr Rauer busy until the opening of the Exposition, provid[ed] [Rose] can get him and his staff over here, establish them, and give them work enough to finance them for not less than two months."[16] Rose responded in the affirmative and was so confident in Rauer's reputation that he advanced him $2,000, which was almost $50,000 in today's relative worth.[17]

Newspapers heralded Rauer's arrival in the United States in June 1914 and claimed that his models would offer visitors to the Panama-Pacific International Exposition an engrossing experience. Allegedly Rauer was going to craft a "human heart so large that visitors may walk through it and watch the pumping of the red and blue blood through the ventricles and auricles, and study the effects on the great life engine, of impurities in the blood, and of fresh air."[18] He was also going to construct "a human eye as large as a bay window, showing the destructive effects of bad factory lighting."[19] Lastly, supposedly, Rauer was going to make "a model of a fever mosquito as large as an ostrich" for Cuba.[20]

While Rauer did craft some models, none were as spectacular as initially promoted. Moreover, the archival record of the IHC indicates that working with Rauer was a complicated and often frustrating endeavor.

The IHC desired an exhibit that would display all phases of hookworm disease and demonstrate the effectiveness of public health campaigns. The aesthetics of the renderings both of the microscopic organism and its manifestation in the human body deeply mattered to the IHC. In order "to reproduce minute details true to life," the IHC believed that Rauer needed to immerse himself in "the heart of an afflicted region."[21] Consequently, the IHC sent Rauer to Wilmington, North Carolina, to work with Charles Wardell Stiles, the director of the RSC.[22] From the start, almost everything went wrong. It probably did not help that Stiles was known to have an "acerbic" temperament.[23]

First, when Rauer arrived in the United States in mid-June, he brought finished products with him. In Germany, he had crafted wax figures in postures of repose. However, the IHC was "not at all anxious to be in possession of wax reliefs with closed eyes and in lying position[s]."[24] These representations did not reflect the reality of the lived experience of hookworm infection in the United States.

Ernst Meyer, the IHC's director of surveys and exhibits, traveled to Wilmington to discuss the situation with Rauer. During this face-to-face conversation, Rauer repeatedly asserted, "Upright cases [of wax] could not be made and had never been made."[25] After this exchange, Meyer returned to his office in Washington, D.C., and interrogated Rauer's claims. After a brief survey, Meyer learned that other artists crafted upright models using plaster of Paris casts to make an initial mold, which they then treated with wax. The effect, Meyer believed, was to "have a certain advantage over figures made solely of wax in that they are not repulsively life-like but are sufficiently so to be thoroughly convincing." Meyer wrote to Rauer explaining his findings. In response, Rauer immediately reversed his previous position.[26]

Although not without some doubts, Meyer asked Rauer to prepare several arms, a foot, a section of skin, and wax reliefs of hookworm cases before and after treatment. Rauer received another $1,000 ($500 upon signing and another $500 upon completion) toward "the cost of preparing the said models" when he signed a contract on June 26, 1914.[27] In an internal memorandum, Meyer expressed hope that the additional money would prevent Rauer from "souring" on his work for the IHC.[28]

With the help of Stiles, Rauer set to work creating realistic reproductions. First, Stiles took him to several homes in Columbus County, after which Stiles believed that "[Rauer] underst[ood] why it was that models lying down were not satisfactory to us."[29] Second, Stiles recruited several young men to work as models, for which they received between $1.50 and $3.00.[30] Although Rauer assured Meyer that he could easily make the reliefs that the IHC desired, the archival records suggest otherwise.

Described as a "famous case in the literature, [Selma Ellis] was desired for modelling."[31] In July 1911, a severely underweight sixteen-year-old Ellis was brought to an RSC county dispensary in North Carolina. The ulcer on his leg was so painful that he was unable to stand.[32] A year later, Stiles presented Ellis and another boy, Luther McPhereson, to the members of the American Public Health Association as a "living comparison of the efficiency of the fight being waged in the South against hookworm disease."[33] Ellis "looked like post-mortem material . . . when [the RSC] discovered him" but here he was "strong and hearty looking" in contrast to McPhereson, who appeared "fair, thin, and waxen of hue."[34] Ellis's celebrity extended beyond the conference when newspapers picked up the story.[35]

On June 2, 1914, Stiles telegraphed Meyer that Rauer's casting procedure had broken open Ellis's ulcer. Stiles advised Meyer to abandon the process "unless some other method [became] possible" as the "ordeal [caused] too much risk."[36] In a longer letter the next day, Stiles recounted what he had witnessed and the unfortunate result.

> [Rauer] first made a cast of the back of Selma Ellis, some of the plaster ran around his shin and as it was taken away it took part of the healed ulcer with it. I immediately insisted that the ulcer be bandaged before the ventral cast was made. After a little argument he consented to this. The second cast was, as I wrote you, a very careless piece of work from my point of view. . . . Selma has been down several times since then to sit as a model, but his ulcer was in such condition that I had to put him to bed yesterday. It is impossible to tell how much damage has been done, and how long he will have to be in bed before the ulcer heals.[37]

Stiles was not alone in objecting to the process. Upon seeing Ellis's injury, two other "cotton mill boys . . . refused to have anything further to do with the matter." Another boy began vomiting before the cast was complete and had to be removed. A fourth boy declined to participate again unless he was paid $100.[38] Similarly, a fifth boy spurned a second sitting, "say[ing] that he can not be hired to go through with it again, as it pulled the hair on his body too much when the cast was taken off."[39]

Despite misgivings, Stiles grudgingly continued to work with Rauer because delays would have complicated matters for the IHC. However, Stiles forced

Rauer to change his process. Instead of placing two-thirds of the body into a
cast at once, Rauer agreed to encase one body part at a time. Rauer also allowed
a physician to remain on site during the procedure. Nevertheless, Stiles was "not
enthusiastically convinced of the ultimate success of [Rauer's] work."[40]

For the next year, Ellis's injuries continued to be an issue for the IHC. The
immediate remedy was to pay Ellis $5.00 "for [his] rough handling by Rauer's
assistants."[41] Stiles also hospitalized Ellis at the U.S. Marine Hospital in North
Carolina and began paying him $12 a month on behalf of the IHC as compensa-
tion for lost wages. Five months after the incident, Ellis was still incapacitated
and appealed to Stiles and Meyer for continued financial support: "I am very
sorry that them germans broke it down . . . and I think they art to pay me untille
it is healed."[42] Rauer, however, never paid Ellis. Only the IHC did.

In a private set of correspondence to Stiles, Meyer wondered for how long
the IHC should remunerate Ellis. Meyer told Stiles in January 1915, "I wish we
were through with this matter."[43] Stiles responded that Ellis had been making
approximately $35.00 a month before his injury, and he warned Meyer, "In my
opinion Selma has ample ground for a lawsuit."[44] Stiles argued, "the Commission is clearly responsible from a moral point of view for taking Selma away
from a position in which he was earning a living and putting him into a condition in which he cannot earn a living."

In May 1915, according to Stiles, Ellis's ulcer was entirely healed and the
IHC ceased its payments.[45] Ellis continued to write Rose, Meyer, and Stiles asking for money. He told them that his leg had "broke down on the lower side
where it healed up last."[46] This time he did not find a sympathetic ear. Writing
to Rose, Stiles argued "that if Selma gets it into his head that he is to be taken
care of the rest of his life no matter what the conditions are, it will be the worst
thing in the world for him."[47] Reflecting middle-class attitudes about deserving and undeserving poor, Stiles believed "there is some moral responsibility
for [Ellis's] loss of time resulting from the accident."[48] He did not think, however, that Ellis deserved a lifetime award. In the end, Ellis was left to fend for
himself.[49]

In addition to the problem of Ellis's injuries, the IHC found itself entangled
in another complication with Rauer: the question of acquiring Rauer additional
work. Rauer was under the impression that Alvin E. Pope had secured him other
contracts. Upon arriving in the United States, however, Rauer confided to Meyer
that he was afraid that Pope was going to "simply leave [him] in the lerch [sic]."[50]
For instance, despite alleged promises from Pope to the contrary, Cuban officials informed Rauer in late June that they would not need his services.[51] Publicly, Pope blamed any lost work on Rauer's delays.[52] Privately, Pope told Meyer

that he was "informed . . . that Dr. Rauer's excitable manners were very annoy-
ing to Dr. Bennett and that they believe this was the sole reason for Cuba refus-
ing to accept the plans." Pope told Meyer that Rauer's "unbusinesslike methods"
would surely make obtaining him other work difficult. Meyer, however, believed
that the IHC was obligated to help Rauer: "he has been brought here upon the
responsibility of the Commission and naturally looks to us to do what we can
for him."[53] As a result, Meyer began writing letters of introduction and making
inquiries for work on Rauer's behalf.

Despite the additional financial allocation Rauer received in June, he continually asked the IHC for more money before he completed the models. When
the IHC did not respond, Rauer began telling stories of woe to third parties, specifically J. B. Gantz, the Secretary of Commissioner General to the Atlantic
States for the Panama-Pacific International Exposition, and Sterling H. Bunnell,
a mechanical engineer.[54] Gantz and Bunnell wrote on behalf of Rauer to Meyer
and Rose.[55] Even Bunnell admitted that perhaps the issue lay with Rauer: "I am
trying to . . . bring some commercial soundness into his affairs."[56] It was unclear
whether Rauer's lack of cash occurred because the onset of World War I prevented him from accessing his German accounts or whether he was incapable
of balancing his books.[57] In looking back on the episode in 1940, John A. Ferrell told H. W. Rose, Wickliffe Rose's son, that "while [he thought Rauer] possessed considerable skill, he was not very orderly in business procedures, and
in one way or another your father and I had to devote considerable time and
effort to concluding the arrangement with him."[58]

Even Meyer's patience wore thin when it looked as if Rauer was going to
stiff the IHC with an outstanding bill from Schieffelin & Company for $69.29.
The invoice was for materials sent to Rauer in June 1914. For the next several
months, Meyer kept forwarding Rauer copies of the bill as they continued to
appear on his desk. Meyer characterized the dispute as an ethical one: "You put
yourself in the position of wishing to escape financial obligation by urging legal
technicalities upon me in return for the readily given assistance to you on the
basis of personal honor and business integrity."[59] Despite promises to pay, Rauer
did not. Instead, Rose paid the bill.[60]

Whatever the IHC's discontent with its financial dealings with Rauer and
its frustration in having to take care of Ellis, it was happy with the results of
Rauer's artistry. As reported in the *Survey*, the International Health Commission's presentation at the Panama-Pacific International Exposition, which
opened in February 1915, was "one of the most frequented of the 'health' or better 'disease' exhibits."[61] The Exposition's International Jury of Awards recognized Rauer with a diploma of honorable mention for the Grand Prize.[62] In

writing a letter of introduction for Rauer, Meyer expressed admiration for Rauer's skill: "So faithfully have details of anatomy and of surface coloring been reproduced that not infrequently visitors to the booth are in doubt as to whether the legs and arms shown in the show case are human flesh and bone or wax."[63]

Rauer's models visualized the symptoms of hookworm disease and its microbial processes of infection. He created a foot to demonstrate "ground itch," the inflammation hookworm larvae caused as they "bore their way through the skin, particularly between the toes."[64] Another model magnified the entrance of the larvae into the body by eighty times. A third model rendered hookworms attaching to the intestine at actual size. Three more models showed the course of infection on a forearm.

In addition to spotlighting the process of infection, Rauer put bodies on display to provide viewers with a holistic image of the disease in different stages. He created an "upright model of a boy 14 years old" to "represent the average case of medium infection." Here there were "no striking symptoms of the disease" but "there [was] a certain pallor and emaciation . . . [and] a slight tendency to 'pot belly.'"[65] In contrast, a different model displayed "emaciation, pallor, pot belly, and aged expression" and another other "show[ed] extreme emaciation, pot belly, aged expression, dwarfing, and retarded development."[66] Rauer also illustrated "angel wings," with a model of "the back of a boy, with shoulder-blades showing prominently."[67] Despite a criticism or two "emanating from women," the fact that the facsimiles were nude went unremarked by the majority of visitors.[68] The IHC's faith in Rauer's expertise to render sterile realism had been realized.

Ellis's leg was also on display in the form of two models representing an ulcer before and after healing. The first model represented "an ulcer in the healing stage," for which Rauer used photographs to construct.[69] The second Rauer described as "the condition of the anemic ulcer three years later." Rauer argued that the "blood spots in [this representation of] the ulcer" were there because "the boy had . . . been working part of the time in the woods and . . . had freshly damaged it."[70] Ellis's injury was made visible to viewers, but the label lied as to its cause.

Rauer attempted to turn his celebrity into a new business.[71] He sent materials to state health officers with letterhead that stated, "Philipp Rauer, Expert in Expositions Organization and Material."[72] He asserted that his work was superlative because he copied actual cases to make his models. By way of example of his painstaking attention to detail, Rauer boasted that senior health officials could use his models to teach a "local health officer the difference between chicken-pox and small-pox in the early stages."[73] In addition to anatomical

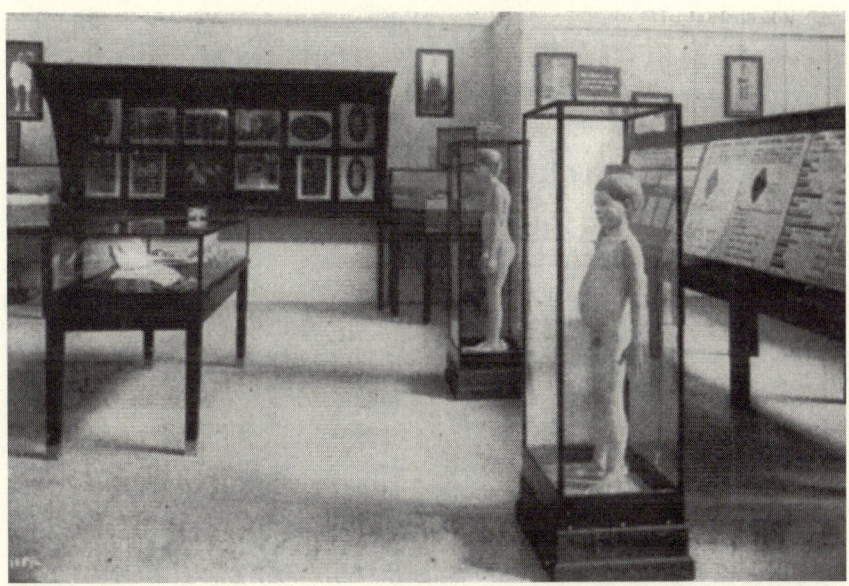

Philipp Rauer's hookworm models on display at the International Health Commission's presentation at the Panama-Pacific International Exposition in San Francisco, California, 1915. Source: *Survey* 34 (July 3, 1915).

models, Rauer maintained that he could make "miniature models of landscapes" and "buildings and engineering structures."[74]

Rauer set up a studio in Hoboken, New Jersey, and developed an affiliation with the Safety Museum in New York.[75] In August 1915, it displayed an exhibit of "Shoes and Feet" that contained many models crafted by Rauer. The purpose was to demonstrate the relationship of "ill-fitting, badly designed footgear" to podiatry problems.[76] Sitting in the window of the museum, consequently, were models of feet with "bunions, corns, and ill-shaped toes."[77] Rauer worked from actual cases to render visuals of "deformed and normal feet" that were "startlingly life-like" in their depiction of "the skin, veins, and coloring."[78] In reporting on the exhibition, the director of the museum, William H. Tolman, recounted an anecdote to illustrate this point: "Excuse me," said a little girl to Tolman, "but would you tell me if those feet in the window are real?" "Certainly," he replied, "but would you mind telling me why you want to know?" "Sure," she said, "it's like this. My mother bet my father that those feet were real and she asked me to find out."[79] According to the reporter, Rauer was, "undoubtedly, the most artistic specialist in this field."[80]

In the late 1910s, Rauer developed a relationship (of what exact nature is unclear) with Permolin Products Company. J. R. Levy incorporated the company in January 1917 for $12,000.[81] In December of that same year, Permolin Products Company increased its capital from $12,000 to $100,000.[82] In 1918, Rauer filed a patent for the "process of producing modeled objects and apparatus for use in connection therewith" and assigned it to the company.[83] Afterward, it seems that Rauer gave up on public health exhibition and began applying his artistic techniques to other applications. An advertisement from the early 1920s, for instance, describes a series of dolls that could be purchased from Permolin.[84]

As the nature of popular health education changed in the twentieth century, it appears that Philipp Rauer's fortunes dissipated. In 1935, he owed P. Heymann $16,637.70.[85] He tried to adapt to these new circumstances by changing his specialty from model making to working in the pharmaceutical industry. In 1941, as president of the Allied Commercial Corporation, he leased a new "one-story industrial building on the north-east corner of Borden Avenue and Thirty-fourth Street, Long Island City," for the "manufacture of chemicals."[86] Ten years later, Rauer was charged with attempting to sell counterfeit Cortisone.[87] The newspaper report described Rauer's office as a "shabby, makeshift affair."[88] Since his arrival in the United States thirty-seven years earlier, his fortunes had fallen very far.

Not all scientific artisans made anatomical models of people; Mica Heidemann made a living sculpting insects. It was not that she was not adept at depicting people. Heidemann created a bust of Charles Darwin for the National Museum in 1889. In 1900, she received a commission to build a statue of Mrs. Louise Pollock, president of the Washington Normal Kindergarten Institute. In 1907, her artistry was requested by the Smithsonian to make a bust of Spencer F. Baird, the institution's second secretary.[89] Instead, it was Mica's husband, Otto Heidemann, a famous entomologist, who influenced her decision to focus her commercial trade on insects.[90]

Otto Heidemann migrated from Germany in 1873 and initially made his living as a wood engraver.[91] He initially set up shop in Baltimore but moved to Washington, D.C., to secure government work in 1876. There he "supplied numerous illustrations for government publications."[92] In 1883, "he was appointed engraver in the United States Department of Agriculture."[93] After engraving insects for fifteen years, he became an expert on the family of the Hemiptera ("an order in the insect world the individuals of which are recognized by the beak") and an assistant entomologist within the department.[94] His path to entomology was typical, as "amateurs and professionals alike would journey by train or trolley for a day or weekend collecting."[95] Heidemann did much of his specimen gathering in western Virginia, and these excursions were a family affair.[96]

Born in 1860, Mica Zester married Otto Heidemann in 1879.[97] She developed a national reputation after the Treasury Department's Bureau of the Public Health Service used her models in its presentation at the St. Louis World's Fair.[98] An article from the *New York Sun* in 1906 suggests that her gender, her artistry, and the nature of her work informed her celebrity. Titled "Making Gigantic Bugs," the newspaper article described her model-making process, the types of insects she crafted, and the purpose. The U.S. Department of Agriculture (USDA) wanted her models to evoke both a visceral and rational response.[99] It also wanted to evoke support for its research and programs designed to foster agricultural productivity.

Heidemann's first step was to take an insect and place it under a microscope to study its "shape and proportions." She then drew a rendering of the insect in the "same proportions" as the intended model. Using steel wire, Heidemann created the "bills, legs, feelers, and sometimes the framework of the body." This skeleton then received a coat of paper mache. Sometimes she used gutta-percha, a rubbery material derived from subtropical trees that could be molded when wet or hot. She used "clay glazed over and then tinted in the natural colors" to re-create worms. She used "fine celluloid" for insect wings. The work was time-consuming: "so delicate is the work that a month may be occupied in finishing a weevil or mosquito." Heidemann preserved her physical and mental health by "work[ing] a few hours at a time and then g[ave] her brain and hands a rest."[100]

Before and after the world's fair, Heidemann found a market for her expertise among states looking to demonstrate the threat of insects on agricultural produce. In 1904, the State Entomologist of Minnesota paid Heidemann eighty-one dollars (approximately $2,000 in today's currency) for "models of injurious insects for use in lectures to farmers."[101] In 1908, the New York State Museum noted in its annual report that it had made "two important additions" to its collections that Heidemann "executed."[102] She made an "enlarged model of the onion fly, showing the egg, maggot puparium, adult fly and an onion infested by maggots." She also made "an enlarged model of the cigar case bearer showing its work upon apple leave [*sic*]."

In 1916, Joseph Y. Porter, Florida's chief health officer, sought Heidemann's help after he learned about her work from the Treasury Department's Bureau of the Public Health Service.[103] In a series of correspondence, Heidemann explained to Porter that she typically made models between seven and twelve inches but could make any size to order. At first, Porter did not quite understand the precise nature of her work and requested a model of a dog and horse; Heidemann informed him that insects were her specialty and she "[did] not make models

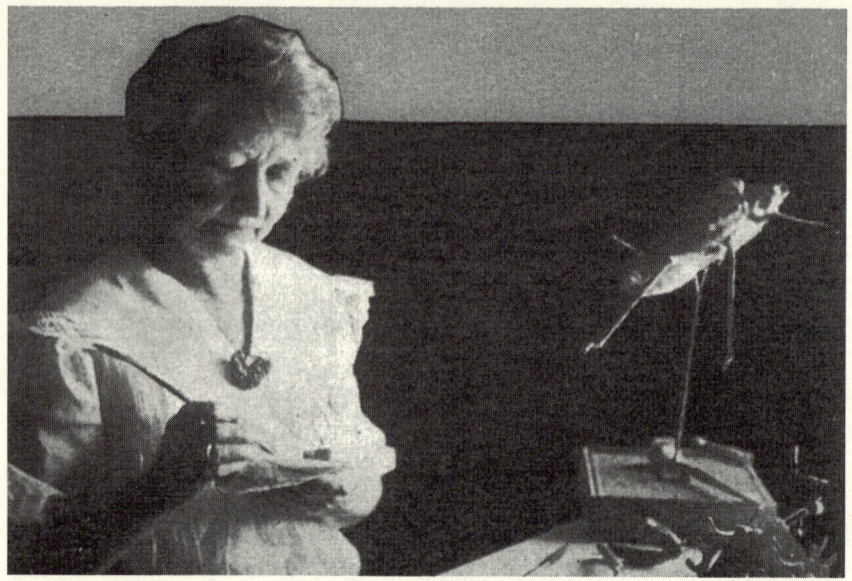

Mica Heidemann at work. Source: *Technical World Magazine* 9, no. 4 (June 1908).
Image Courtesy of University of Michigan Library.

of Mammals." Porter then asked her to make a male and female cattle tick, three
different mosquitoes, and a rat flea. The combined price was $410 (a little more
than $9,000 today).[104]

In late November 1916, Otto Heidemann died suddenly.[105] Afterward, it
does not appear that Heidemann continued with her work. Within a few years,
she moved to Schenectady, New York, where she found residence in her niece's
home.[106]

For a time, artists like Rauer and Heidemann found a niche market and were
able to make the most of it. Their models displayed public health threats in ways
that their patrons desired: realistic and sterile. However, their expertise was
expensive, and their personalities were sometimes cantankerous. Moreover, the
customized nature of their work entailed painstaking hours to complete. When
a cost-effective competitor, the Educational Exhibition Company owned and run
by Gardner T. Swarts, arrived on the scene, it captured the market.

Mass Production: Gardner T. Swarts Jr. and the Educational Exhibition Company

Gardner T. Swarts Jr., the son of a very prominent pioneer in public health reform
in the United States, unintentionally began the process of standardizing public

health exhibits.[107] Foreseeing a financial opportunity, somewhere in the late summer of 1909, twenty-four-year-old Swarts founded the Educational Exhibition Company to "design and equip educational exhibits of all kinds," in particular, "everything necessary for traveling exhibits of public health."[108] Located in Providence, Rhode Island, the Educational Exhibition Company began providing health-minded reform organizations and state officials throughout the nation with models, posters, photographs, and charts. Swarts's company explains why exhibits throughout the United States often looked the same; his models circulated through the market.

When he started his business, Swarts did not intend to make a career out making public health exhibits. After graduating from Harvard in 1908, Swarts became a civil engineer. In that capacity, he found immediate employment in public health organizations, translating the specifics of sanitation as it related to tuberculosis into layman terms. Swarts worked as a "demonstrator" (today what museum professionals refer to as a docent) for the Rhode Island State Exhibit at the International Congress on Tuberculosis in September 1908. He secured a similar position at the International Exhibit on Tuberculosis during its run from November 1908 to January 1909 in New York City. Afterward, he found full-time employment with Samuel M. Gray, who was Providence's city engineer. Swarts took a few leaves of absence during his hire, always to work at expositions (the "Boston 1915" and a few produced by the Rhode Island State Board of Tuberculosis).

In 1912, Swarts realized that his "side line" business needed his full attention. He convinced a former Harvard classmate, Robert F. Gowen, to join him in partnership. Four years later, Swarts took full control of the company's management.[109]

While Swarts had worked at large exhibitions, his company created exhibits geared toward smaller spaces and intended to be temporary. Swarts's company produced materials anticipating that they would be used in public libraries, clubs, lodges, railroad stations, and schools. He also envisioned small displays placed in transitory spaces such as store windows, department store restrooms, doctors' offices, hotel lobbies, office building arcades, and corridors. He intended to reach people in the spaces of life's pauses.

Between 1910 and 1917, Swarts produced at least five catalogs that detailed his company's products and offered advice.[110] Rather than mere lists, most of the catalogs read as short books. Swarts included lengthy descriptions and instructions to sell his merchandise. He called his third catalog a "textbook."[111] Exhibiting public health might have been popular, but according to Swarts's catalogs, it was not simple.

The layout was a major issue. According to Swarts, exhibit attendees tended to construct individual paths through exhibit space much to the chagrin of exhibit makers. In response to this dilemma, Swarts asserted that he was the "originator of the zig-zag, or maze system of planning the layout of an exhibit, requiring spectators to view every part of the exhibit in its proper order."[112] One of the reasons, he argued, that his "panorama" exhibit was so exciting was that no one could "begin at the wrong end of it and work backwards as he may be looking in the usual picture-hung exhibition."[113] Swarts, perhaps based on his experience as a docent, did not trust visitors' ability to be autodidactic.

He was also very concerned about lettering. He believed in clean lines and clear text. Swarts critiqued the Fourth International Congress on School Hygiene as a partial failure due to its "slovenly lettering."[114] He argued that "great care should be used to prohibit verbosity and the use of inferior lettering and insignificantly small photographs."[115] Swarts advocated that lettering be "as large as possible so it may be read across a wide hall."[116] He discussed typeface and wording in detail, providing an example of contrasts.[117] He was a major proponent of using "mottoes or aphorism" in conveying ideas to audiences.

For those who worried that exhibit making was a complicated process, Swarts assured potential customers of the operational ease of his products. The crates he used to ship the exhibits, for instance, transformed into the skeleton upon which to hang the displays. This rendered construction knowledge superfluous. In many locales, electricity was still a novelty. Consequently, Swarts emphasized the user-friendly aspects of his materials: "No electrical knowledge is necessary to operate these illusions beyond that required to screw a plug into a lamp socket."[118] All of Swarts's objects were inorganic, and he warned against using pathological specimens unless they were "few in number and well selected."[119] Photographs, artifact reproductions, and illustrations offered those unfamiliar with scientific laboratory techniques a stable and consistent presentation.

To bring drama to what otherwise might feel like static messages, Swarts emphasized the theatrical nature of a number of his creations. He used sound and light to draw attention. For instance, he argued, "people will often listen to a phonograph who would not let a man say a word to them."[120] The contrast rooms, he suggested, were "something entirely new and are well adapted to holding the attention of the public as an element of mystery is attached to them."[121] He created two scenes. The first exhibit piece showed a dirty room replaced by a clean one. A second piece depicted visitors to a drinking fountain. In the opening scene, a "careless consumptive" drank from a common cup. After a few seconds of darkness, Swarts's model relit, and a mother could be seen holding that same cup up to her child's lips.[122] Swarts also produced several macabre objects for display. Dolls turned into skeletons.[123] Babies in cradles dropped down dark holes and were replaced with gravestones.[124]

Judging by Florida's experience, Swarts's salesmanship was compelling. Joseph Y. Porter, Florida's chief health officer, purchased some objects in developing an exhibit to display at the American Public Health Association's (APHA's) annual meeting in 1914.[125] According to Porter, this was the first time the APHA departed from their "ordinary routine discussion of papers."[126] Swarts was particularly interested in Florida's business because he knew "it would be to [his] advantage to have [his work] present at the meeting."[127] Initially, Swarts hoped to attend, but he had so many orders for the upcoming Panama-Pacific International Exposition that he had to beg off from making a personal appearance.[128]

Out of the Educational Exhibition Company's catalog, Porter purchased a farmyard well model, rural fly model (that showed flies "traveling from the barnyard and privy vault to the dining room"), gross fly stick pins, a baby graveyard model, a contrast room illusion, death rate illusion, a small patent medicine bottle, twelve Red Cross shields, and a comic face with mirror mouth.[129] Porter also ordered a few "portable exhibits": a type E exhibit on a house fly, a type E exhibit on tuberculosis, one Bell Death Rate Sign "similar to your cat. No. 515 but with a new copy for 'Preventable Diseases,'" and one type E exhibit on babies.[130] The combination of exhibits influenced almost all of a person's five senses. Where the flashing bulbs and graphic images captured people's sight, the Bell Death Rate Sign demanded people listen.

The company also built to order, and Porter asked Swarts to create an artesian well and sewage disposal model and a model of an Imhoff tank. In negotiating the specifics, Swarts and Porter conversed about how to modify these models to enhance their "realism." Swarts suggested "placing a scenic background behind the [sewage] model." He also suggested adding a "background illustrating several houses indicating a village in the distance" for the Imhoff tank because the "tank is designed for a population of one thousand (1000) people and it w[ould] look rather inappropriate we believe to show a tank of this size as though it was attached only to a single house." Swarts estimated the cost for these models at $579.00, which would be close to $13,000 today.[131]

In the 1910s, Gardner T. Swarts found a market for mass-produced public health models and displays. Although not everything was as realistic as Heidemann and Rauer's work, Swarts offered a wide variety of materials that depicted various aspects of public health. Comparatively, while Swarts's artistry was not awe-inspiring, he did embed elements of drama.[132] At the same time that Swarts was building his business, a nonprofit organization providing advice on best practices evolved alongside Swarts's commercial enterprise. Similar to Rauer, Heidemann, and Swarts, the Russell Sage Foundation believed that artistry mattered in producing effective communication.

Setting Standards: The Russell Sage Foundation

In 1912, the Russell Sage Foundation (RSF) hired Evart G. Routzahn to serve as the associate director for the Foundation's newly established Department of Surveys and Exhibits. He held this position for twenty-two years, until his retirement in 1934.[133] In that period, he became the dominant voice in the etiquette of popular public health education.

According to Shelby M. Harrison, the director of the department, the RSF's goal was to provide "wider and more effective dissemination of information aimed to promote the welfare of individuals and families, the community, and social work organizations laboring to improve social conditions."[134] The RSF's underlying belief was that if you made the information "more interesting and easy to understand," "its popular spread could be more rapid."[135] Harrison was responsible for overseeing the department and focusing on surveys. Routzahn was responsible for professionalizing the production of exhibits.[136]

Routzahn began his career in social work at the YMCA in Dayton, Ohio, and later moved to Chicago.[137] It was there that he attracted the attention of H. H. Jacobs, president of the Wisconsin Anti-Tuberculosis Association. Routzahn's "flair for visual expression, a term which was utterly unknown in those days, attracted the notice of a number of people."[138] The National Tuberculosis Association hired Routzahn to supervise its traveling exhibit from 1906 to 1912.[139] In doing so, he became the Association's first full-time salaried employee.[140] He simultaneously assisted in the creation of an exhibit for the Sixth International Congress on Tuberculosis in Washington, D.C., in 1908.[141]

Routzahn explained his philosophy on the use of exhibits for publicity in the *Survey* in 1909. He argued that while "the tuberculosis exhibition is in no sense a revolutionary force: it does not overthrow things; it will not bring an immediate reorganization of the universe," it was "expected to awaken interest, to impart information, to lead to activity, and to suggest work to be done and plans for doing it."[142] The goal was to provide information to "an intelligently interested and awakened constituency."[143] He believed that an effective exhibit must provide an audience with "something to get people to look at, something to explain what people are looking at, and something to get people to talk after they have looked."[144] He warned against displaying anything too sensational that could lead audiences to "inaccurate deductions." He also warned that "undue sensationalism" could prove to be "unpleasant or obnoxious to any considerable number of people."[145] Similar to Swarts, Routzahn rejected the use of pathological materials for popular public health education, contending that specimens "too nearly correspond to that of the patent medicine advertisement."[146] Lastly, while Routzahn acknowledged the importance of popular health education for all audiences, he believed that the ultimate aim should be to reach those in places of power: "The immediate need is to win the leaders, people who do things, those who rent houses, pay wages, fill offices, teach school, preach or lead in churches or otherwise manage affairs. Win the leaders and the rank and file can be reached."[147]

The RSF created the Department of Surveys and Exhibits to act as a clearinghouse for information and as a consultant on best practices. Harrison was an expert on statistics and surveys. Routzahn brought "the fruits of six years' experience in the exhibit campaigns of the National Tuberculosis Association conducted in more than forty cities of Canada, Mexico, and the United States."[148]

One of Routzahn's first actions in his new position was to send a survey to national associations engaged in philanthropic work. In explaining why he needed people to respond, he wrote, "No other problem in exhibition technique, however, seems to present more perplexities" than the "sizes and materials" that should be "used in mounting exhibits."[149] The questions asked about whether the organization in question had a policy for exhibit making on background sizes and units displayed, type of board to use ("comp board, beaver board, rock board, etc"), and what kind of framing the organization used.[150]

Routzahn also continued to act as a consultant to organizations throughout the nation. It was in this capacity that Routzahn became acquainted with Mary B. Swain, who would become his professional and personal partner. Swain grew up in Milwaukee and received a BA from the University of Wisconsin in 1902. After teaching high school English for five years, she spent a year at the University of Chicago specializing in sociology. Afterward, Swain took a position with the Juvenile Protective Association of Chicago. In 1913, she organized an exhibit in Peoria, Illinois, titled "Cycle of Child Life" and asked for help from Routzahn's office. According to the newspapers, Routzahn and Swain "work[ed] in close co-operation."[151] Although the exact timing is unclear, Swain relocated to Washington, D.C., that same year, where she created an organization called the Children's Council, which was a social welfare agency for children.[152] Shortly afterward, the RSF appointed her to its staff. Five years later, Swain and Routzahn married.

Together, the Routzahns, who were described as "indefatigable," became synonymous with popular public health education.[153] From the RSF "they [ran] an information bureau, an employment exchange, a museum of models and horrible examples, and a lighthouse of counsel and guidance."[154] Evart Rout-zahn was never without opinions. By way of example, in 1914, he told Ernst Meyer of Rockefeller's International Health Commission (IHC) that while the exposition of safety and sanitation was "vastly superior" to that of the previous year, Routzahn still found "the majority of the exhibitors fail[ed] to utilize up to date exhibit technique in the proper development and interpretation of their exhibits."[155] The following year, he suggested to J. A. Farrell of the IHC that "one of the things which I think needs to be developed is the large easily portable illustration, which can be seen by the audience in a good sized room."[156]

Despite complications, the Routzahns did not waiver from favoring exhibits as a mechanism for communication over printed tracts. Their reasoning was myriad. They argued that an exhibition, by its nature, "attract[ed] the attention of people who would not go to a lecture or read a pamphlet."[157] The brevity of exhibits, they contended, was attractive especially to men who "get no further than the baseball news or the comic page in the evening paper."[158] According to the Routzahns, the community nature of exhibits prompted group conversations. They also argued that exhibits provided exhibit makers a more tangible sense of audience because they could count the number of people who visited. Lastly, the Routzahns believed the use of docents was particularly advantageous because "explainer[s]" could meet "people in small groups," which afforded them "an opportunity for valuable personal contacts, such as printed reports, and even lectures do not offer." The Routzahns explained, "The visitor can ask [the docent] questions which, in the case of the printed page, he cannot ask the author."[159]

Despite the advantages, the Routzahns warned against misapplications of this form of publicity. They argued that every exhibit needed to have a purpose from its onset. Filling up space, they maintained, was not a legitimate reason to install an exhibit. They also suggested that the effectiveness of providing scientific explanations to justify public health policies depended upon the audience. They believed, for instance, that teaching "tenement mothers to keep flies out [with] detailed scientific or technical charts demonstrating the method in which flies carry disease germs w[ould] not be very convincing to them." Instead, the Routzahns contended that the more useful message would be to demonstrate very simply and practically how windows c[ould] be screened at small expense, or how as an alternative it [was] at least possible to keep flies away from the baby and from the food."[160] As they explained in 1919, "while health is something that everyone wants, the desire to follow advice for getting it is usually in conflict with personal and group habits, also with desires that are cultivated by those who sell foods, clothing, recreation, and stimulants and with the misinformation about easy preventives and cures offered by dealers in patent medicines."[161]

The goal of the public health exhibit was to appeal in a format "that c[ould] win against these handicaps."[162] Evart Routzahn offered six ways in which an exhibit could serve as a mechanism to engender public health:

> 1. Education of individuals in personal hygiene so that they will not catch or spread disease and so that they may improve their own health and that of their families. 2. Advertising the services of nurses, clinics, dispensaries, health centers and hospitals. 3. Gaining the co-operation of special groups, as tenement dwellers, restaurant proprietors, and storekeepers, so that the work of inspection may be made easier and more effective. 4. Gaining the support of voters for legislative programs on public health and sanitation. 5. Appealing for financial support of private health agencies. 6. Organization of volunteer co-operation to extend the work of the health agency.[163]

After six years of providing individual consultations and accumulating information, the Routzahns published a book on the subject, *The ABC of Exhibit Planning*. Despite the many years of organizations using visual displays, the Routzahns believed that exhibits still tended to be "clumsy tool[s], awkwardly used."[164] A review in the *Survey* told potential readers that it covered "media and techniques."[165] In addition to "dos," the book advised against "devices that look good, but have been proven futile and even dangerous."[166] The power of the book, the reviewer argued, lay in its "origin in experience, not in theory."[167] In addition to the text, the Routzahns included numerous photographs to illustrate principles in practice.

Similar to the points Evart Routzahn had made in 1909 about exhibitions related to tuberculosis, the Routzahns maintained that the most critical aspect of exhibit production began with "visualize[ing] your audience."[168] Exhibit makers needed to know if the public health policies their exhibit proposed would come into cultural and economic conflict with visitors: "We want to know also whether the reform or the thing proposed upsets old customs or perhaps affects their pocketbooks."[169] Understanding the visitor also meant knowing what would impair their desire or ability to attend in both cultural and practical terms. As examples, the Routzahns discussed the case of Jews and workers: "If we want to reach mothers, many of whom are Jewish, we won't choose a Hebrew holiday nor set up the booths in the Sunday school rooms of a church. If the exhibit is to interest working people, we won't have all the special features in the mornings and afternoons."[170]

In providing conceptual help, the Routzahns discussed the merits of different types of exhibits: the community exhibition, the convention exhibition, train exhibits, traveling campaign exhibits, loan exhibits, the "drop-in" or casual exhibit, exhibits at fairs, and museums of social welfare. They did not advocate for one type over another. However, they did have a list of warnings for most. The community exhibition might contain too much diversity in its material and cause "confusion of ideas in the minds of visitors."[171] Convention exhibits suffered from being overcrowded. As for train exhibits, the Routzahns argued that their novelty had worn off. Drop-in or casual exhibits, they contended, lost their effectiveness if their presentation appeared "stale."[172]

Exhibits differed from the printed pamphlets because exhibits melded visual and textual materials together. Still, some aspects overlapped between the two strategies. On technique, the Routzahns agreed with Swarts's assessment that lettering mattered. The Routzahns objected to panels that used text that was too small or in all capitals. Doing so, they argued, impeded comprehension.[173]

Another impediment to communication, according to the Routzahns, was overcomplicating the exhibit's errand. They advocated sticking to singular messages. They argued that displays needed to focus on "one idea at a time."[174] They believed that commercial advertisers instinctively understood this advice. Distilling the message, they argued, increased the impact of the impression.

In addition to conceptual advice, the Routzahns discussed practical concerns about exhibit creation. They argued for less text, the use of harmonious colors, and large images. They felt that photographs, for instance, worked best when at least 11 by 14 inches in size.[175] They also supported "manipulating the details of photographs to obtain striking results or to make a picture fit into a particular space or design," which they argued was similar to "newspaper practice."[176] The Routzahns did not see photographs as inviolate sources of evidence but rather as pieces of propaganda for public health policy.[177] They supported the use of three-dimensional models, as long as their purpose was clear. They also warned about making contrast rooms either "too good" or "too bad," arguing that the visitor would not be able to identify with exaggerations.

At the end of their book, in an appendix section, the Routzahns provided potential exhibit makers with a series of planning documents. They created a list of budget items to consider, which included materials and labor. They offered advice to pass on to volunteer committees whose job it might be to help or create an exhibit. This advice included suggestions on whom to add on what committees and ideas on how to delegate the various types of work (from publicity to construction). The third appendix was the outline used for the Stamford Baby Week Exhibit so that readers could see how the theory was put into practice.

Lastly, the Routzahns provided "an example of an explainer's talk." The Routzahns believed that people who served as "explainers" served as useful supplements to an exhibit by stimulating conversation.

The art of exhibit making, according to the Routzahns, entailed more than the panels, photographs, posters, graphs, models, and explainers. Without a central argument and without tailoring to a particular audience, they contended, an exhibit failed to promote public health. Their 234-page book provided guidance, but it was clear that creating a compelling display of public health was not a simple endeavor.

In 1934, the Department of Surveys and Exhibits underwent a name change and became the Consultant in Social Work Interpretation. Evart Routzahn believed that "this [wa]s a change in name only and d[id] not affect the nature of the work done." He explained that "the exhibit, earlier recognized as an important tool for public education, ha[d] for some time been absorbed into the broader field of educational publicity in the Department's studies."[178] Nevertheless, in hindsight, it is hard to not see this as one marker of the end of the general popularity of exhibits to promote public health public policy. The same year as the name change, Evart Routzahn retired. Mary Routzahn carried on her work for another ten years focusing on publicity in general rather than exhibits in particular.

Conclusion

The art of exhibiting public health in the early twentieth century opened up business opportunities as well as prompted discussion about best practices. Individual artists found a market for their skill in visualizing disease and threats to health. Rauer and Heidemann's experiences speak to the possibilities and limits that existed for the scientific artisan. Sensing the prospects, Swarts created a company to sell premade products to health departments and reform organizations throughout the nation. His success explains why so many exhibits throughout the country looked similar; they were the same. The plethora of exhibition led to the Russell Sage Foundation committing funds to develop a department to serve as a clearinghouse of information and a mechanism to promote best practices. The Routzahns collected and shared information on the success and failures of public health exhibition. In combination, the art of popular public health education became standardized. Despite the advice available, executing professional visual displays for popular public health education appears to have remained a conundrum for reformers and officials throughout the nation.

Chapter 3

Health Trains

An Experiment in Traveling Exhibits

In 1913, a reporter from the *Detroit Evening News-Tribune* watched a young woman enter a railroad car at Detroit's Union Station that was fitted with a display on public health. Inside, the woman studied a series of charts on baby care while holding her own fretful "little shaver of about six months."[1] In front of her were two charts on appropriate clothing for summer. On one side was a smiling child in the "slimsiest of summer garments." On the other side was a picture of a very fancy dressed infant howling. According to the reporter, the mother's "cheeks reddened and her eyes grew heavy with self-reproaching tears." She discreetly removed her own child's "lace trimmed bonnet, with blue baby ribbon insertion, a white dress, hand-embroidered, stockings neatly knit, and white kid bootees." With a sigh, her child stopped crying and the woman departed from the stuffy train. Michigan's health officials argued that her reaction "ma[de] us feel that all our effort was not in vain."[2] Although social mores dictated dressing up for an outing, the mother identified her baby's body with the one in the public health display and changed her behavior accordingly.

In the early twentieth century, state health officials throughout the United States hoped to engender financial and moral support for public health through a new vehicle for popular education: the health train. By taking a railroad car, or two, and installing an exhibit of three-dimensional models, photographs, charts, and, in some instances, microbial specimens, public health officials presented messages about disease prevention to thousands of people. The train's advent as an instrument for education dovetailed with the embracement of bacteriology by state boards of health.[3] Health officials believed health trains would be particularly useful for reaching rural audiences because conditions on the farm especially mattered in theories about the transmission of tuberculosis and typhoid fever from rural producers to urban consumers.[4] An analysis of three health trains—the first, California; the longest lasting, Louisiana; and one of Louisiana's imitators, Florida—demonstrates how officials educated mass audiences about the importance of sanitation as a deterrent to the spread of contagious diseases.[5] Ultimately, however, politicians' misgivings about the financial expense of these traveling exhibits and the absence of statistical information on the train's ability to change individual health behaviors caused the train's appeal as a technique for public health instruction to wane.

Initiation: The California Sanitation Car

In 1907, Newell K. Foster, the secretary of the California State Board of Health, traveled to Washington, D.C., to attend a meeting of the U.S. Public Health and Marine Hospital Service with the State and Territorial Boards of Health. Afterward, Foster journeyed to view various educational exhibitions. (He did not leave a record as to why.) First, he traveled to Jamestown, Virginia, where he believed the famed traveling American Tuberculosis Exhibition was on display. Originally opened at the American Museum of Natural History in New York in 1905, the American Tuberculosis Exhibition was the first large-scale public health exhibit built to travel.[6] After thousands thronged to see it in New York, the exhibit was shipped to Boston, Philadelphia, and Chicago. After that, it intermittingly continued to be displayed.

When Foster got to Jamestown, the exhibit was still sitting sealed up in its 110 crates. The exhibit managers "kindly unpacked some for [him], but little could be learned, as they could not be seen to advantage."[7] Afterward, Foster traveled to New York City, where he looked at exhibits sponsored by the Committee for the Prevention of Tuberculosis. He also spoke with the organization's secretary, Paul Kennaday, to get some "pointers" on how to use visuals in public health education.[8] Upon Foster's return to California, he authorized the fabrication of exhibits for the state fair in 1908 and began discussions about deploying "a railroad car to demonstrate sanitary problems."[9]

Although it is not clear where Foster got the idea for a train car, it is probable that he read about the recent use of railroad cars for other educational efforts. In 1904, Perry Greeley Holden, professor of agronomy at the Iowa Agricultural College, decided to create an extension class to reach farmers throughout the state.[10] He persuaded the Rock Island and Burlington railroads to allow him to send four cars equipped with educational exhibits and classroom space along its routes. It was nicknamed the "Corn Gospel Train," and newspapers covered its escapades.[11]

California's officials similarly believed that a health train could be an efficient, durable mechanism to educate the public on best sanitary practices within domestic, commercial, and industrial spaces in both urban and rural areas to prevent the spread of contagious disease. The California public constituted over two million residents, of which approximately 60 percent lived in urban areas.[12] Health officials viewed rural and urban health as interconnected because urban consumers increasingly relied on rural sources for their food.[13] The general press supported their opinion. The *Los Angeles Times* stated, for instance, "it is in the rural population that is constantly furnishing the cities with typhoid fever and with milk from tubercular cows."[14] The Country Life Commission, an initiative by President Theodore Roosevelt to study rural life in the hopes of modernizing it, also supported this view. The commission argued, "Infection may be spread from farms to cities in the streams and also in the milk, meat, and other farm products."[15] Consequently, California's health train addressed preventive strategies for common communicable diseases for both rural and urban audiences.

Scholars often focus on the significant influence of private philanthropy in the development of public health infrastructure, particularly in the South.[16] California's officials also relied on private investment to a certain extent. In putting together California's train, Foster worked primarily with William Freeman Snow, who was a professor of preventive medicine at Stanford University. The two had traveled together to the International Tuberculosis Congress in Washington in 1908.[17] Upon their return, they entered into discussions with Colby Rucker, an assistant surgeon of the U.S. Public Health and Marine Hospital Service. These conversations built upon an earlier collaboration between the California Board of Health and the federal government to combat plague in San Francisco in 1903.[18] Rucker, in turn, worked to convince the Southern Pacific Railroad Company to donate a car.[19] In asking business leaders to defray the cost of civic education, Rucker was asking them to participate in the type of philanthropic activity articulated by Andrew Carnegie about the obligation of "the man of Wealth" to distribute surplus funds for "the most beneficial results for the community."[20] When Foster became too ill to continue as secretary of the California State Board of Health in June 1909, Snow was elected unanimously to be his successor.[21]

Snow used "a corps of students" to construct a variety of displays to immerse the visitor to the sixty-foot train in medical messages.[22] Images of the inside of the train indicate that Snow placed dioramas in glass cases along both walls of the railroad car (he had removed the seats). Charts and graphs covered the walls

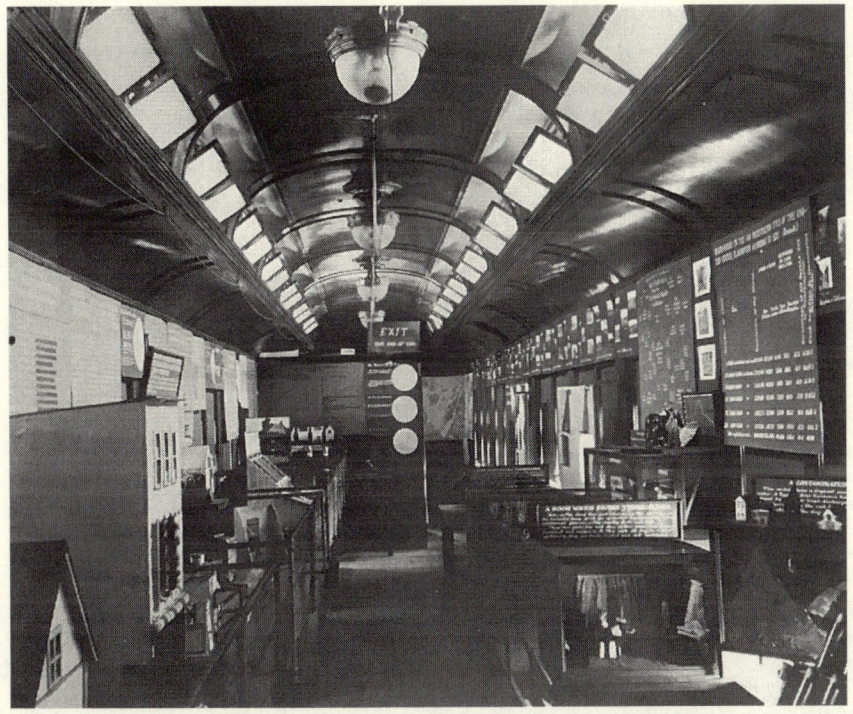

Inside California's Sanitation Car. Source: H. O. Jenkins, "A Traveling Sanitation Exhibit Directed by the State Board of Health of California in 1909," California State Library. Photograph by Shauna Mulvihill.

and most of the tops of the windows. Snow left the bottom half of the windows open to allow for ventilation and light. At night, officials illuminated the car with gas lamps.

Although Snow included information about malaria, smallpox, typhoid fever, and other communicable diseases, tuberculosis was the primary focus of the exhibit.[23] The emphasis on tuberculosis reflected the enormity of this public health problem in California. Public health officials described "tuberculosis as the most serious single disease citizens of the State have to combat . . . los[ing] annually 5,000 citizens."[24] Although health officials increasingly blamed migrants, especially Mexicans, they recognized that the bacillus did not discriminate.[25] Snow included "several hundred photographs, showing conditions favoring tuberculosis."[26] He also used dioramas to depict tuberculosis as a threat in both urban and rural domestic living arrangements. Lastly, he installed a display wherein a bell rang every three minutes to represent the estimated 175,000 annual national deaths from tuberculosis.[27]

Unlike tuberculosis exhibits produced in the Northeast or Midwest, however, officials did not provide materials in multiple languages. Officials might have felt justified in limiting their efforts because only 3.7 percent of California's population over the age of twenty-one in 1910 was illiterate in English.[28] Illiteracy, however, was much higher among foreign-born whites and racial minorities.[29] Thus, the omission of bilingual materials suggests that officials' target audience was native-born whites.

Unfortunately, only a few images survive of either the interior of the train or individual objects.[30] From this limited pool of visual evidence, it appears that officials placed large posters with magnified pictures of various microbes labeled "the germ of bubonic plague," syphilis, gonorrhea, and leprosy above a corresponding diorama. In turn, the dioramas rendered information about the importance of sanitation in dramatic juxtapositions. The model of the dairy, for instance, was split into two halves. Snow's students painted one side white, added a cooling house with screened windows, and left the ground free from dirt. They left the other side unpainted and displayed manure in the yard and stables.

Similarly, the diorama related to plague prevention showed two versions of the same home. Students installed measures to discourage rats and squirrels from taking up residence on one side of the diorama and left garbage and litter throughout the yard on the opposite side. These creations encoded refuse as the primary vehicle for disease transmission and sanitation as the remedy.

Although Snow designed the models to be approximations, he was concerned about conveying "realism." He went beyond employing artistic optical illusions to make materials lifelike. In the "country home," for instance, he instructed the students to glue "real flies" that they had "killed" to "the back-house walls and kitchen fence and also to a fine wire which [was] stretched from the back-house window directly thru the open kitchen door to the dining table."[31] While the presentation disregarded laws of proportion, it highlighted the role of flies as vectors of disease.

In another instance of compromised authenticity, Snow placed a doll on an attic bed to represent a diseased person in his or her rural residence. Although the interpretive label read "Tuberculosis in the Farm House," Snow told officials on the train that they could describe the "bed-ridden doll . . . as either a typhoid or tuberculosis patient . . . to illustrate the principles of contagion in the household."[32] The solution to either ailment, officials argued, was better sanitation.

While there was faith in the use of objects to educate, it was not total. California's health officials feared that the public might not take away the messages

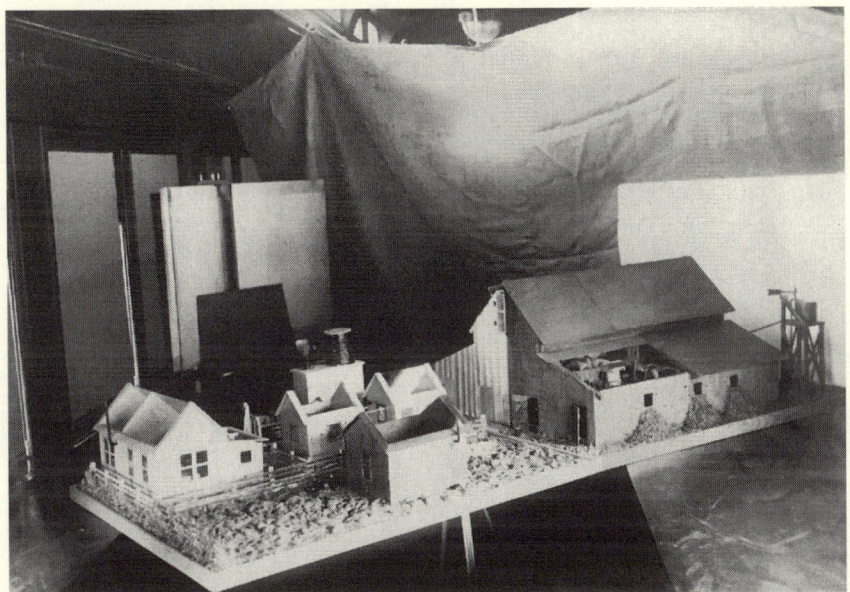

The "Bad" Dairy Barn. Source: H. O. Jenkins, "A Traveling Sanitation Exhibit Directed by the State Board of Health of California in 1909," California State Library. Photograph by Shauna Mulvihill.

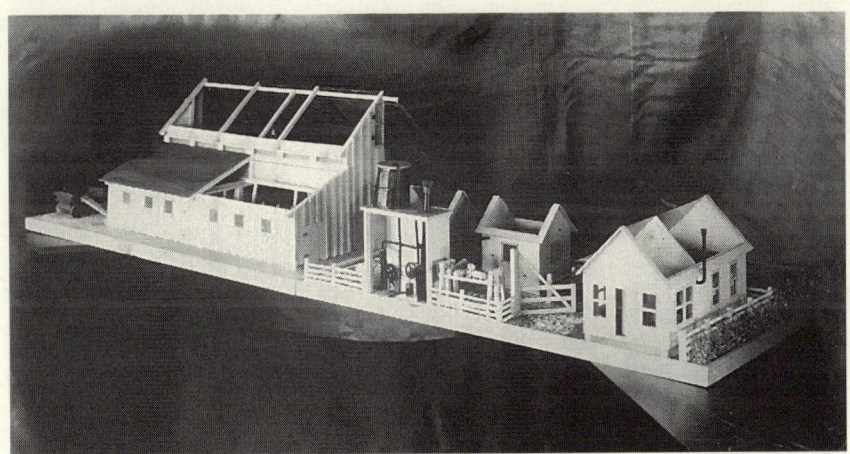

The "Good" Dairy Barn. Source: H. O. Jenkins, "A Traveling Sanitation Exhibit Directed by the State Board of Health of California in 1909," California State Library. Photograph by Shauna Mulvihill.

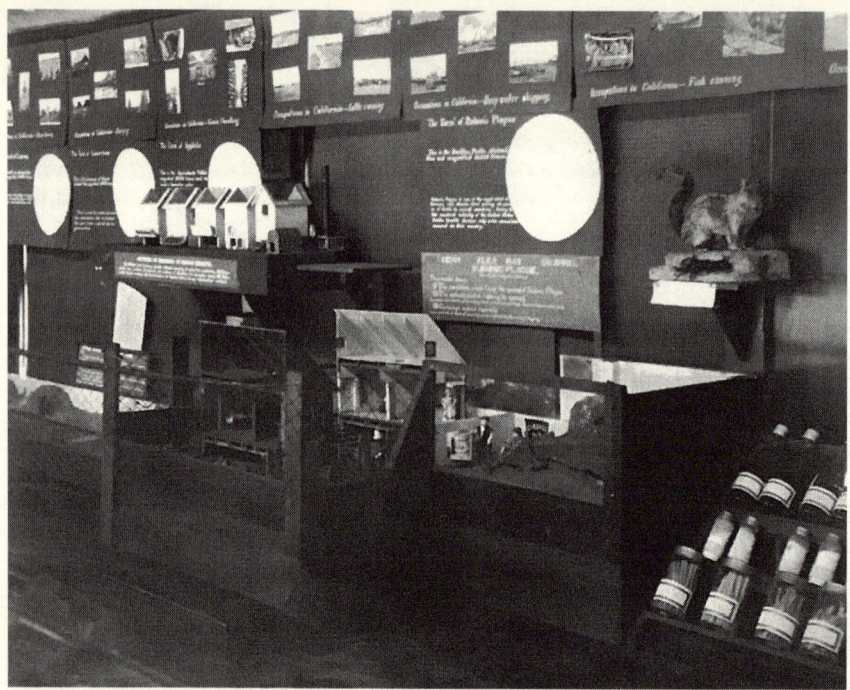

"Contagious Diseases Explained." Source: H. O. Jenkins, "A Traveling Sanitation Exhibit Directed by the State Board of Health of California in 1909," California State Library. Photograph by Shauna Mulvihill.

they intended to impart. As a result, they employed a docent to accompany the train whose job it was to "give plain, practical talks on the methods of preventing disease."[33] Officials emphasized that these talks be straight "to the point and brief."[34] Besides brevity, the train's personnel used lantern-slide lectures at night to combine education with entertainment. If a room was unavailable, they hung a curtain and proceeded with an outdoor stereopticon lecture.[35]

With an enormous banner attached to the train's side, it began its tour in Palo Alto in March 1909 and then made its way to San Jose, the Joaquin Valley, San Francisco, the Monterey Bay region, and finally Southern California.[36] Nothing in the state's literature about its venture suggests that officials had any particular ethnic or racial group in mind when deciding where to take the train. The main concern of officials appears to have been volume and, by all accounts, the train was successful in attracting audiences. In Los Angeles, "hundreds visited the health exhibit car."[37] A later estimate put the figure at "thousands."[38] The newspaper noted that in San Francisco, "men and women from every station in life, clubwomen and laundry girls, physicians and brick layers, farmers

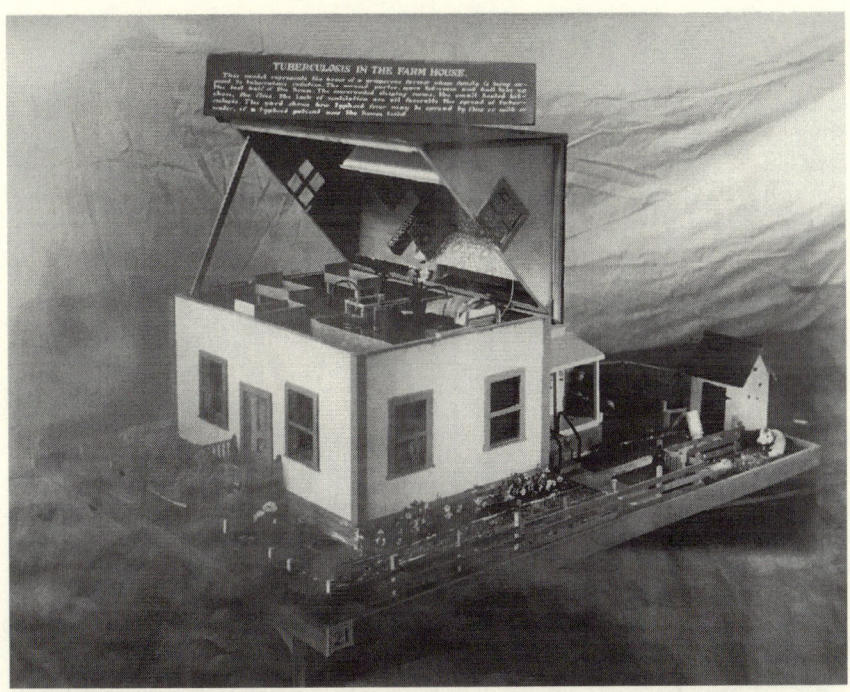

"Tuberculosis in the Farm House." Source: H. O. Jenkins, "A Traveling Sanitation Exhibit Directed by the State Board of Health of California in 1909," California State Library. Photograph by Shauna Mulvihill.

and businessmen" came to see the car.[39] When the train's journey was completed in February 1910, officials estimated that the train had attracted 80,000 visitors in the ninety-two places that it had stopped.[40]

What did California's health officials believe to be the impact of the health train? H. O. Jenkins admitted that "direct and definite results from such a work as this [were] hard to ascertain."[41] Overall, the board argued that the "greatest good that the Car ha[d] done was no doubt, to start people to talking and thinking about the needs of sanitary precautions and to bring them more in sympathy with public health work."[42] The train, consequently, served most importantly as propaganda.

In June 1910, the California State Board of Health believed that there was the support to continue running the train: "numerous requests for its continuance were read."[43] A month later, the board of health's opinion shifted in the opposite direction. Bowing to pressure from the state's governor, James Gillett, the board voted to terminate the train. The February minutes read, "The continuance of the Sanitation Car was brought up, and the Secretary reported on

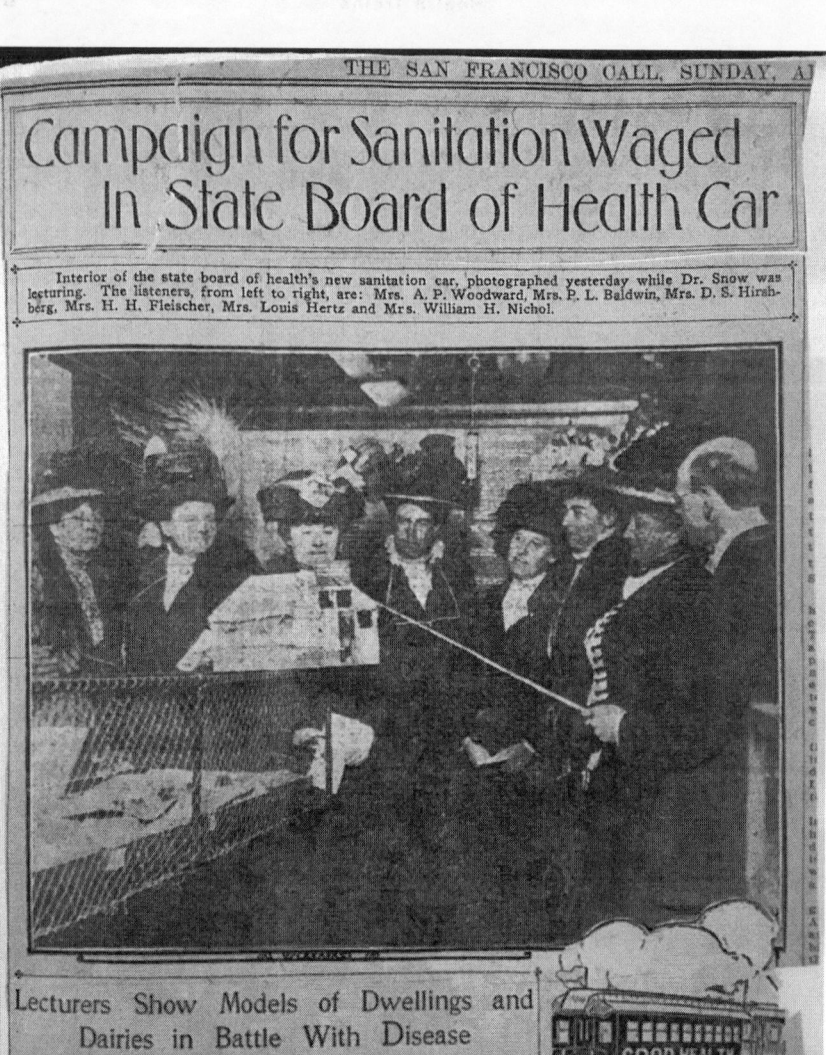

Campaign for Sanitation Waged In State Board of Health Car

Interior of the state board of health's new sanitation car, photographed yesterday while Dr. Snow was lecturing. The listeners, from left to right, are: Mrs. A. P. Woodward, Mrs. P. L. Baldwin, Mrs. D. S. Hirshberg, Mrs. H. H. Fleischer, Mrs. Louis Hertz and Mrs. William H. Nichol.

Lecturers Show Models of Dwellings and Dairies in Battle With Disease

Men and women from every station to life, clubwomen and laundry girls, physicians and brick layers, farmers and businessmen, thronged the California sanitation exhibit car at the Third and Townsend streets depot yesterday, listening to the lectures with

cisc supplied the car and transportation and yesterday it rolled into San Francisco, and the educational movement was opened.

CLUBWOMEN VISIT CAR

The plan met with instantaneous success. The car was thronged all day

GOOD HEALTH

Docents explained the California Sanitation Car's displays to a variety of audiences. In this case, William Snow lectured a group of clubwomen. Source: H. O. Jenkins, "A Traveling Sanitation Exhibit Directed by the State Board of Health of California in 1909," California State Library. Photograph by Shauna Mulvihill.

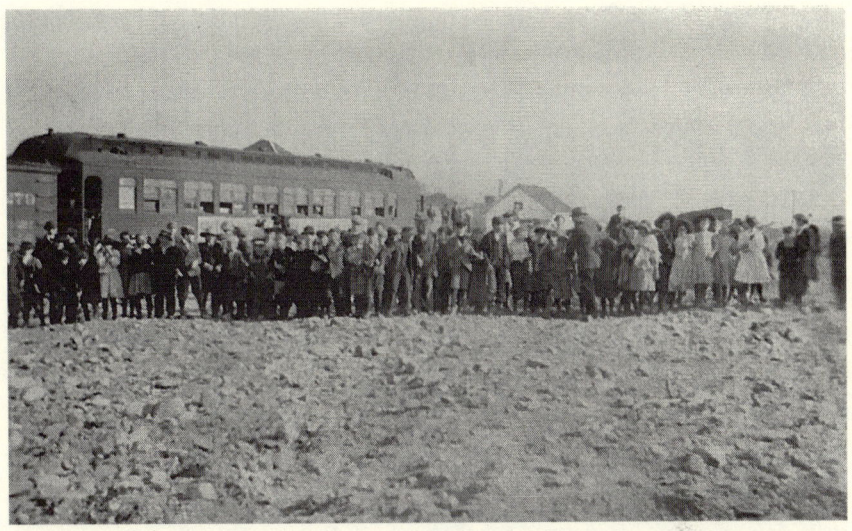

Schoolchildren were a captive audience for California's health officials. Here, those from Hayward pose for a group photograph before entering the train. Source: H. O. Jenkins, "A Traveling Sanitation Exhibit Directed by the State Board of Health of California in 1909," California State Library. Photograph by Shauna Mulvihill.

the Governor's attitude toward the continuation of this work. Moved by Dr. Standsbury, seconded by Dr. Ainsworth, that the car be dispensed with for the present. Carried."[44] The board did not document the precise reason for Gillett's objection.[45] It is possible that he was unhappy with the expense of the train. Initially, the "Governor agreed in conference on July 15th to approve the movements of the car for six months at a total expense not to exceed $2,400."[46] The state's annual financial report, however, listed the sanitation car's expense as $3,352.63.[47] While the board initially left room to revisit the topic, it did not resurrect the train.[48]

Transforming an Experiment into a Model: The Louisiana Health Train

Just as California decommissioned its health train, Oscar Dowling, the president of the Louisiana State Board of Health, decided to expand upon the concept.[49] First, he retrofitted his railroad cars with electricity. Second, he viewed this project as a permanent one, and his highly publicized endeavor ended up lasting the longest of any state, running from 1910 to 1928. Third, he outpaced all others in attracting an audience. In the train's first two years, when it ran a total of 396 days, Dowling counted 308,378 visitors at the 391 locations the train stopped.[50] Dowling's venture caught the attention of the state boards of health in Michigan,

Iowa, Colorado, Kentucky, Virginia, Maryland, and Florida and continued to hold an attraction for state boards of health into the early 1930s.[51] Although the health trains were a national phenomenon for a time, the continuous use of them in Louisiana and intermittent use in Florida, Kentucky, Virginia, Arkansas, Texas, and Georgia gives a southern bent to the narrative.

The story of Louisiana's health train is a critical articulation of the dynamics of public health in the New South, where changing notions about efficiency, entrepreneurship, and industrialization simultaneously intersected and evaded long-standing norms about race relations. Contemporary conversations about the New South focused on messages of investment and racial harmony.[52] The gospel articulated by the health trains embodied the optimism of reinvention and made presentations about health in relation to developing southern economies. At the same time, health officials obeyed and implemented racial segregation. Unlike the West, where it appears that California's officials did not envision racial minorities as an audience for the train, southern health officials made sure to include African Americans, albeit at separate times.

Questions of rural health in the South were particularly crucial for southern public health officials because much of the South's population lived in rural areas well into the twentieth century.[53] In 1910, the year that Dowling put his plan into action, 70 percent of the state's population lived in rural areas.[54] County health departments, however, did not exist until the 1910s and did not grow in significant number until the 1930s.[55] Instead, responsibility for rural health in the South fell to state boards of health.[56] Their primary focus in the nineteenth century was suppressing epidemics of yellow fever.[57] In the twentieth century, confirmation that water and sewage served as transmission routes for dangerous microbes created new opportunities for authorities to advocate for large projects of civic infrastructure.[58] Also, the identification of new diseases, such as hookworm, made individual rural lavatory constructions civic questions. State officials often made use of philanthropy to study and respond to these new issues, of which the Rockefeller Sanitation Commission for the Eradication of Hookworm Disease played particular importance.

The Rockefeller Sanitation Commission, which functioned from 1909 to 1914, left "a network of state and local public health agencies [in the South] in its wake."[59] Another significant result of the Commission's efforts was the creation of a coherent message between public health officials and educators about the relationship of reform to modernity.[60] Additionally, the Commission's integration of exhibits into its dispensary activities played a critical role in attracting participants and fostered anticipations of "the spectacular."[61]

Health trains functioned in similar ways to the Commission's demonstrations. First, an aura of wonder surrounded the health train's arrival. In small towns with limited opportunities for entertainment, its appearance was comparable to the circus.[62] Second, the train's exhibits justified investment in civic programs for public health, which included campaigns to change hygienic practices. Furthermore, in Louisiana, the Rockefeller Sanitation Commission used the health train to carry out its mission.[63]

The launching of Louisiana's train coincided with the onset of the state's work with the Rockefeller Sanitation Commission. Sidney D. Porter, one of the state's sanitary inspectors, was appointed to work under the auspices of the Commission in October 1910. He "equip[ed] [himself] with [a] microscope, lantern, and slides" and began surveying the extent of hookworm throughout the state.[64] A few weeks later, Dowling appointed him "Director of the campaign for the eradication of Hookworm disease" and put him on the train as it began its journey. The train allowed Porter to collect samples from almost every parish and confirmed the prevalence of the disease.[65] Riding the train also allowed him to expand his public education efforts. On board, the exhibit contained both models of "sanitary closets" and "specimens of hookworms and other intestinal parasites" for public viewing.[66] Porter targeted physicians with a different type of education. Victor F. Carey, the "microscopist in charge of the train," prepared slides of "hookworm eggs" to then give to physicians along the route "who had microscopes."[67] In doing so, Porter participated in standardizing exchanges of bacteriological knowledge among medical professionals.

Establishing and maintaining a health train was a costly endeavor. Dowling recounted in his annual report that he had difficulty obtaining the proper materials, especially expensive railroad cars. Apparently, "the presidents of the railroad companies laughed at the Utopian dream."[68] They would not lend him two railroad cars when "the supply was limited and no new ones obtainable."[69] Eventually, he was able to convince the president and general manager of the Queen and Crescent Route, the superintendent of the New Orleans and Northeastern Railroad [sic], and the superintendent of the Vicksburg, Shreveport, and Pacific Railroad to donate two cars temporarily.[70] (After the train's success, Dowling purchased three Pullman cars: two for exhibits and one for staff.) In addition to needing a loan to begin his project, Dowling required free passage on the rail lines. At the end of the first fiscal year, Dowling estimated that the 10,623 miles the train traveled throughout Louisiana would have cost the state $6,287.17 if the railroad companies had charged for their use.[71]

Where Dowling did not appear to encounter difficulty was in establishing a relationship with Tulane University. Tulane's medical faculty donated twenty jars of pathological specimens, including eight of tuberculosis-diseased organs and twelve healthy ones for comparison.[72] The school also lent Dowling "sections of lungs in different stages of pneumonia, tuberculosis, and a diseased heart interior."[73] Dowling enhanced these displays by adding a model of an eye, nose, throat, and ear. He also put on display samples of "tuberculins and antitoxins, and other bacteriological projects."[74] The specimens and models made the relationship between human anatomy and disease visible. However, they sometimes proved too graphic. "A mother" from Patterson, Louisiana, wrote to the editor of the *Times-Democrat*, "I wish to protest against the promiscuous exhibition of dismembered parts of the human body to show disease. While these 'specimens' may be beautiful to the young M.D., they give a real shock to the nervous system of a young child."[75]

Taking advantage of having two cars, Dowling categorized Louisiana's exhibit into five "lessons," through which "the main lesson of each [was] apparent even to the casual observer."[76] Dowling's goal was to "present, graphically, simple health truths."[77] The categories were preventable diseases, pure food, sanitary necessities, model household sanitary equipment, and personal hygiene and community sanitation."[78] There was also an antituberculosis exhibit and the hookworm disease exhibit. Visitors could view a model dairy, slaughterhouse, school desk, and "heating apparatus" for schools and churches. They could see what "modern bathroom fixtures" looked like as well as the latest technology in "disinfectant sweepers, dust cloths and vacuum cleaners." Dowling also offered visitors "transparent views of defective water supply" for dairies, markets, and yards.[79] All of Louisiana's trains always carried expert docents because, according to Dowling, "the science of health [was] so new [that the public could] not be expected to know its principles."[80] While many of the objects appear to have been similar to California's display, Dowling's use of electricity was a significant departure.

Dowling believed that the use of electricity was especially useful in arousing interest because rural residents in the state (and region) generally lacked this amenity. Some of these electrical displays tended toward the macabre. A ghoulish model, for instance, lowered a scythe every twenty seconds on the head of a baby to represent infant mortality rates.[81] Electrically powered flashlights proved to be another dramatic way to dramatize death. Louisiana's train confronted visitors with an exhibit that used a "flashlight showing number of deaths of children" from "ignorance and dirt."[82] In addition to the exhibits, officials used electricity to play three films at night: "The Man Who Learned," "The Red Cross Seal," and "The Fly Pest."[83] Most of the time, Dowling showed these films from the train because the majority of towns did not have an electrically wired public space large enough for screenings.[84]

Unlike California's health officials who did not write about visitors by race or ethnicity, health officials in Louisiana discussed their engagement with African Americans. They did so because they believed that "this race of people is both potentially and actually more capable of disseminating disease among the white people than are the white people among themselves."[85] Employing a strategy of temporal segregation, officials in the South made special arrangements for African Americans to visit the train.[86] They also played the movies at night separately and arranged discrete lectures.[87] In connection with the train's visit, officials asked African American ministers to inform their congregations that a "special lecture will be delivered to them on the subject of sanitation by a trained negro physician who is specially fitted for this work."[88] In providing "special" talks, white public health officials helped perpetuate the notion that African Americans' hygiene habits put society at risk. At the same time, however, this fear prompted public health officials to allow African Americans access to what they believed was cutting-edge public health education.[89]

Newspapers circulated information about the Louisiana health train widely throughout the United States.[90] Perhaps the Louisiana health train's most glamorous advertisement was its transcontinental trip to the annual meeting of the American Medical Association (AMA) held in June 1911 in Los Angeles. Dowling spiffed up the cars by writing "Louisiana State Board of Health Exhibit" in gold letters on the outside. The 5,000-mile trip included stops in Houston, San Antonio, El Paso, Santa Barbara, San Francisco, Salt Lake City, Ogden, Cheyenne, Denver, Omaha, Fort Dodge, Waterloo, Dubuque, Rockford, Chicago, Kankakee, Champaign, and Memphis.[91] In taking the train to Los Angeles, Dowling included materials related to Louisiana's industries and resources. According to Dowling, "a pamphlet was prepared setting forth temperature records, low death and morbidity rates, controllability of endemic diseases and excellence of climatic conditions."[92] Thus, the train functioned as a promotion to business investors in addition to being an instrument for public health education.

There is evidence of a few cynics amid all the hoopla. Writing a letter to the editor of the *Macon Telegraph*, one individual wrote, "The trouble with the Louisiana health train is that the people who go to see it [were] the ones who [were] hygienic anyhow."[93] In Dowling's 1913 report to the state legislature, he acknowledged, "The eradication of mosquitoes has not yet taken so great a hold [because] many people are skeptical as to results of measures recommended."[94] Moreover, he only counted "twenty communities, since 1911, [as] hav[ing] improved their water supply."[95] In addition to these markers of doubt, Dowling found himself subject to a lawsuit.

In November 1914, the health train visited Chattanooga, Tennessee, home of the Chattanooga Medicine Company owned by J. A. and Z. C. Patten Jr. The company's claim to fame was an elixir, the Wine of Cardui. The Patten family had sold the mixture as "the standard remedy for female weakness for years" with great success.[96] Upon learning that the train displayed a poster that attacked the product, the Pattens sued Dowling for libel and claimed $25,000.00 in damages.[97] The exhibited material, which had been created by the AMA, suggested that the majority of the concoction was beer and whiskey.[98] The poster characterized Wine of Cardui as a "fraudulent alcoholic nostrum."[99] For two weeks in February 1916, the U.S. District Court at Chattanooga heard the case. After two of the jurors became sick, the suit ended in a mistrial and was never reopened.[100] A few months later, a similar case against the AMA resulted in a guilty verdict but an award of only a single penny.[101] In these two cases, it does not appear that the general public necessarily agreed with public health officials or the AMA's assessment of the ineffectiveness of patent medicines.[102] Nonetheless, the lawsuit did not dim Dowling's faith in the power of persuasion.

While Dowling theoretically could exert state power over intrastate affairs, he recognized that his best hope of convincing the public to support public health policies was to engage in a campaign of encouragement. Stopping in the various towns, Dowling used the train to highlight each locale's problems but left it to local officials and the public to clean up their communities.[103] He argued that the train was useful because "the logical and immediate outcome of the health exhibit train was a general clean-up day in almost every town visited."[104] Dowling summarized the results: "improved water supply; more adequate sanitary service; an awakened consciousness of the necessity of inspection of food and sanitary environment; a better understanding of the necessity for boards of health and health officers; better service in care of public buildings; and a keener appreciation of the danger of infectious and contagious diseases."[105] He believed that the "result of the health propaganda by means of the cars . . . [was] the awakening of a public health conscience."[106]

While Louisiana's health train ran for a much greater length of time than any other state, its fate was tied to its health officers. Dowling found success as the state's leading health official until Huey Long took office in 1928.[107] Long perceived Dowling's longevity as evidence of corruption and ousted him from office.[108] Dowling contested his removal in court, but he did not win.[109] Under new management, the state board of health discontinued the health train.

Following in Louisiana's Tracks: The Florida Health Train

Florida's senior public health official, Joseph Y. Porter Sr., did not immediately become enamored with the idea of copying his neighbor's experiment.[110] Instead, it took a failure with a different traveling exhibit to push him to attempt the grander scheme. Even then, the Florida health train ran for only two years, 1916 until 1918. Moreover, officials put the train into storage during the summer months because the "intense heat" made it "unbearable" to either visit or operate the cars.[111] (Why they had a more difficult time then Louisianians on this accord is unclear.) Florida's effort at replicating Dowling's experiment demonstrates the difficulties in implementing a health train.

When the American Public Health Association (APHA) decided to hold its annual meeting in Jacksonville, Florida, in December 1914, the organization decided to depart for the first time from its "ordinary routine discussion of papers" and include exhibits. Porter seized the opportunity to procure state funds to create a semipermanent display.[112] He directed his employees to "gather together, as a partial health exhibit, certain explanatory information in the shape of panels, texts, models and electrical devices bearing upon sanitary principles in health management and disease suppression, thus aiding in the general plan of education in sanitary principles."[113] While Porter created the exhibit to demonstrate the state's achievements to other professionals, he had already determined that afterward, he would modify the display into a traveling exhibit to send to county fairs, schools, and auditoriums. Hence, what he created for professionalization became used for popular public education.

To enhance Florida's exhibit, Porter purchased some objects from Gardner T. Swarts Jr., the son of a prominent pioneer in public health reform in the United States. Swarts founded the Educational Exhibition Company to "design and equip educational exhibits of all kinds," in particular, "everything necessary for traveling exhibits of public health."[114] Located in Providence, Rhode Island, Swarts was particularly interested in Florida's business because he knew "it would be to [his] advantage to have [his work] present at the meeting of the American Public Health Association."[115] However, Swarts had so many orders for the Panama-Pacific Exposition in 1915 that he had to beg off from making a personal appearance at the APHA conference.[116]

Out of the Educational Exhibition Company's catalog, Porter purchased a combination of items to influence almost all of a person's five senses. Where the flashing bulbs and graphic images captured people's sight, the Bell Death Rate Sign demanded people listen: "At each toll of this bell someone dies of a *preventable disease* in the United States. 600,000 every year, 1,650 every day, 69 every hour, More than one a Minute These Deaths are *Unnecessary!*" For longer pondering, he secured a farmyard well model, a rural fly model that showed flies "traveling from the barnyard and privy vault to the dining room," a "baby graveyard," a "contrast room illusion," and a "death rate illusion."[117] Similar to the displays on both the California and Louisiana trains, Florida's exhibit advocated the simplicity of sanitary practice.

After the APHA conference, Porter provided the "Educational Health Exhibit" to any organization, municipal or private, that could provide "suitable space for its installation."[118] Porter advised those who wished to bring the exhibit to their city that the exhibition required between 2,000 and 2,500 square feet and "at least 4 electrical connections."[119] Judging by pictures, the display barely fit into a large auditorium.[120] Tall vertical posters attached to panels covered every inch of wall space. Three-dimensional dioramas and objects adorned tables throughout the hall.

In its first year, the Florida exhibit traveled to four different large fairs: Sanford during the Seminole County Fair, Orlando during the Orange County Fair, Tampa during Gasparilla Carnival, and Lakeland during the Polk County Fair. According to Porter, these were "seven of the largest cities of the state."[121] Those running the Seminole County Fair began asking for the exhibit before it was even displayed at the American Public Health Association meeting.[122] The exhibit also traveled to an additional seven smaller urban areas: Ocala, Palatka, Pensacola, Tallahassee (where it stayed for the entire month of April while the state legislature was in session), Melbourne, Fort Pierce, and Miami. Some cities requested the exhibit but did not receive it. St. Augustine's assistant health officer, Maurice E. Heck, wanted the exhibition because he believed it "w[ould] do more than any one thing to bring about a change of heart in this community" where the residents "ha[d] been rather indifferent towards the State Board of Health."[123] Porter denied Heck's request because of scheduling conflicts.[124]

Florida's health officers proclaimed the exhibit a triumph of influence. After visiting the exhibit in Ocala, for instance, local schoolchildren at the town's primary school (which was for white children), with the help of their teachers, began to collect pictures and create labels to produce their own health exhibits.[125] Also, health officials estimated that approximately 40,000 visitors passed through the exhibit in Tampa during that city's annual festival.[126]

While officials believed that the "Educational Health Exhibit" proved useful, they also found it to be expensive and cumbersome to move. For instance, Porter asked the Southern Express Company to reduce the price of transport from a dollar to a quarter per one hundred pounds. Otherwise, he argued, he would be forced to terminate the program.[127] (The exhibit consisted of two trunks and twenty-one boxes, which totaled 5,000 pounds.[128]) Five months after the exhibit began to travel, Porter felt that its transportation by express caused damage to the displays, which were costly to fix.[129] Also, although "the exhibit c[ould] easily be mounted ready for display in less than one day's time," Porter determined that lugging the exhibit to small towns was particularly problematic because it was "impossible to find a hall of a size to accommodate" it.[130]

By placing the exhibit on a train, Porter believed the board of health could bring public health education to "the remotest rural districts, where it is most needed."[131] This was no small task in Florida, where 64 percent of the state's population was living in a rural area in 1920.[132] (Unlike Louisiana's reports about its outreach efforts to African Americans, nothing in Florida's records indicated whether the state made efforts to reach African Americans.) Porter argued that if he had a train, he could bring the exhibit to between thirty to fifty towns every month instead of the current circumstance of six to eight. Porter did not come to this determination alone. Some states had already followed Louisiana's example and created health trains, albeit running them usually for a month or two.

Although Florida had a more extensive state-supported public health program than other southern states, Porter hesitated to act on his own in creating a health train.[133] Porter felt it necessary to procure specific authority from the state legislature before proceeding to purchase the train cars. He enlisted the aid of Dowling in his lobbying efforts.

Louisiana's health train made its first appearance in Florida at the 1914 annual meeting of the American Public Health Association. Held in Jacksonville, Florida, Dowling had sent the health train. Porter asked Dowling to return with the train during Florida's legislative session in April 1915, a request that Dowling obliged.[134] Porter must have been reasonably confident that he could convince the state to support his endeavor because he opened discussions with the Pullman Company about acquiring and modifying a train for Florida before the legislative session commenced.[135]

The state legislature considered Porter's request in conjunction with some different public health questions in 1915. Out of seven bills, the state legislature approved six.[136] Schools needed to provide adequate "facilities for nature's conveniences"; businesses needed to screen windows and doors in areas of food preparation and service; restaurants could not serve raw meat for consumption; butchers needed to cover their products for sale; all privies (private and public) located within incorporated towns needed to be fly-proofed. Failure to follow these laws resulted in a penalty, although it was not very weighty. Transgression was a misdemeanor, and the sentence for conviction could not exceed fifty dollars. Still, the state board of health was proud of these laws. In its monthly journal, the board included a Charles Van Osten cartoon in which he depicted these laws as a brick wall that kept out the monsters of disease. The second brick closest to the top was the Exhibit Train Law.[137] Upon its passage, Dowling sent a letter of congratulation to Porter.[138]

Florida's exhibits followed a similar pattern of organization to Dowling's. Porter had separate sections for tuberculosis, contagious diseases, laboratory work, and laws. He recycled the material from his traveling exhibit and, as far as the archival record shows, did not produce anything new for the health train. What was different was that he attempted to impose a linear order on the material. In addition to marking an entrance and exit, visitors were encouraged to follow a particular path through the two cars. At least one visitor, however, did not believe that there was any route to follow.[139]

Trying to control the visitors' experience was not exceptional. Porter's exhibit followed many of the recommendations made by the Russell Sage Foundation's (RSF's) Department of Surveys and Exhibits, which that organization had founded in 1912 to gather and disseminate information about exhibit methodology and practice.[140] Upon hearing about Florida's interest in creating a health train, the associate director, Evart G. Routzahn, wrote Porter with suggestions. Routzahn emphatically believed that health officials should place materials aboard a health train "entirely in the center of the car" to maximize fresh air and light from the windows, as well as to prevent visitors from missing anything.[141] From the pictures, it does not appear that Porter followed this exact formula in all the cars, but he did in most.[142]

Although Porter often declared the experiment a success, there was evidence of dissent. In Florida, D. R. Fisher, a shipper of oranges, grapefruit, tangerines, and ferns from Pierson, wrote a letter to the editor of the *Free Press*, which was published out of Jacksonville. Signing his letter "A Citizen," Fisher described his visit to the train in negative terms. He characterized the exhibits as looking "antiquated and grimy" as if "possibly some of our officials were present at the 'Eden Musee' auction."[143] (In referencing the recent demise of one of the most famous nineteenth-century museums in New York City, whose wax exhibits became obsolete objects of popular amusement, Fisher injected a bit of sarcasm into his critique.[144]) Afterward, the editor of the *Free Press* decided to require all authors to sign their names when expressing disapproval.[145]

Around the same time, the *Bradford County Times* published a more disparaging assessment of Florida's health train. The editor objected to the state spending money on the train instead of providing more social services for the indigent. In particular, the editor called for the distribution of free typhoid fever

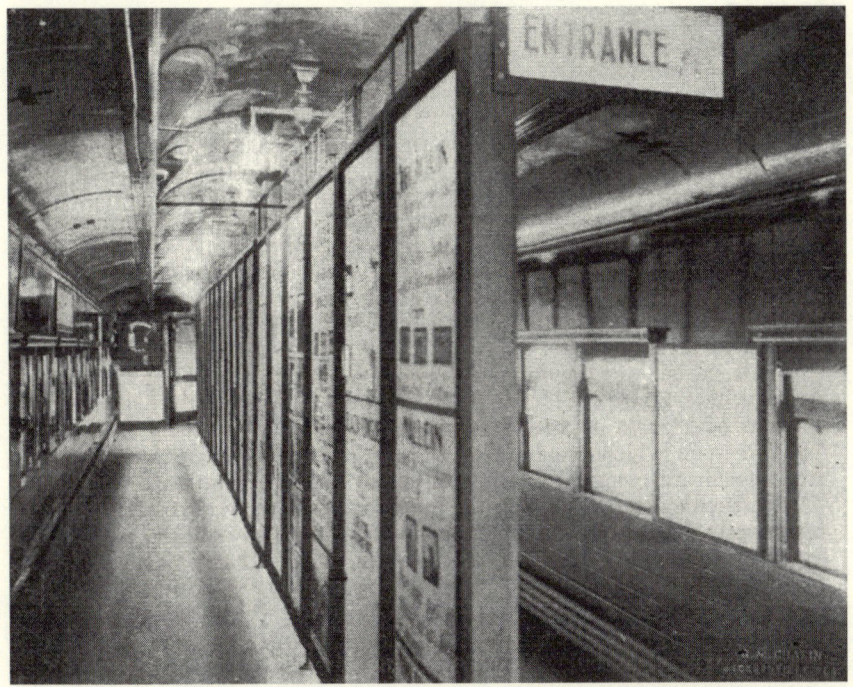

Florida's health officials posted an "entrance" sign to guide a visitor's path.
Source: *Health Notes* 11, no. 1 (January 1916), State Library of Florida.

serum. The condemnation raised the issue of class conflict: "What in the Sam
Hill does a Florida Cracker care for a Pullman train full of bugs and pictures when
his child is on its death bed with a case of typhoid. . . . Give us a Board of Health
for the common people and not the rich who have nothing to do but inspect
Pullman trains out of idle curiosity."[146] Porter responded that the state board of
health provided free vaccinations for typhoid, diphtheria, and tetanus antitoxin.
He ended his rebuttal by stating that the train was "intended to reach people of
all classes."[147]

Although Porter never expressed doubt about the effectiveness of the health
train for public health education, his official reports suggested that the train's
displays did not necessarily result in changed behavior. In rural areas, health
officials maintained that constructing a modern "sanitary privy" was essential
for combatting hookworm. Those who visited the train viewed examples of
human-waste disposal systems for homes and businesses. They could also experience this modernity by taking advantage of the public toilet provided.[148]
However, Porter noted that it had been "so difficult . . . to secure the cooperation of the people" in carrying out these types of projects at their homes that

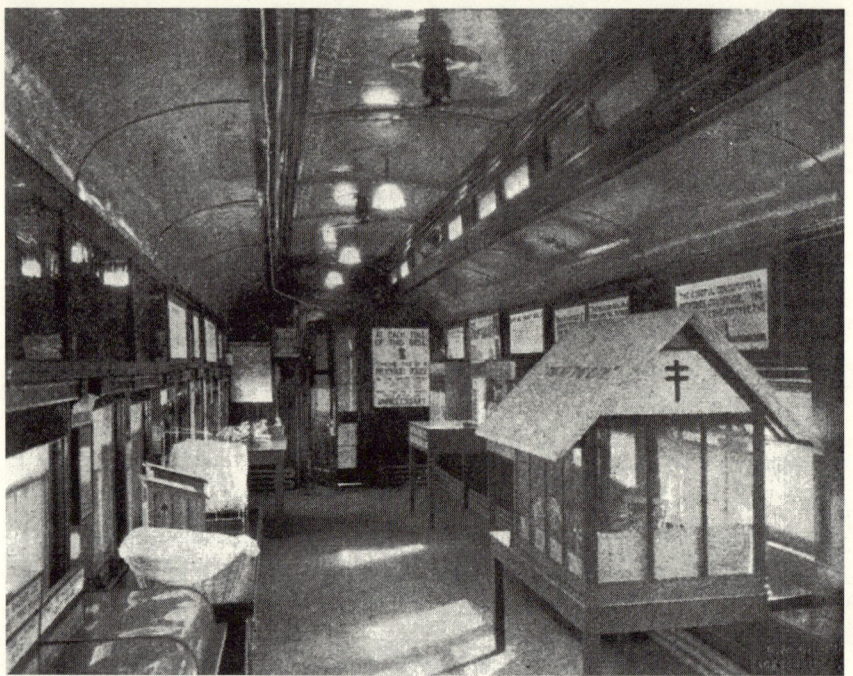

Inside the Florida Health Train. Source: *Health Notes* 11, no. 1 (January 1916), State Library of Florida.

"activities along this line ha[d] been discontinued."[149] Dissemination of information did not guarantee progress in public health.

Despite the critics, state officials were optimistic that they had embarked on a successful strategy. One of Florida's public health nurses, Mrs. F. A. Scott, said, "If we did not meet some people who appreciate our efforts for their benefit, our zeal, and enthusiasm would not last long."[150] On January 19, 1916, Frank J. Fearnside, the president of Florida's board of health, wrote Porter that he believed that the train was a winner: "Everybody I talk to about it seems to think that it is one of the greatest things that the Board has ever done for the general health to the people."[151] Nevertheless, Florida's train experienced a reversal of fortune similar to that of California's and Louisiana's.

Twelve months after Fearnside's declaration, the first glimmer that the Florida train was in political trouble appeared. State board of health member, C. J. Memminger, asked Porter for a detailed explanation so that he could respond to "a certain amount of adverse criticism as to action of our Board in purchase and use of the Health Train."[152] In compiling the data, Porter was worried because the first mathematical accounting created by his assistant showed that "there [was] very little difference between the cost of the exhibit in train service and freight and express."[153] Porter instructed his assistant to redo the document and to "be exceedingly careful to set forth the length of time that the exhibit was operated by freight and express, with attendants traveling expenses, and the same length of service performed by the train."[154] In particular, he wanted the cost of the "purchase of models" and officials' salaries eliminated. He argued that "the same expense to the board is had whether [the official is] in office or on the train . . . , so I do not think that should be included one way or the other."[155] After reading the report, Memminger believed that Porter's detailed analysis demonstrated the efficiency with which the train was run.[156] Nonetheless, once Porter resigned his position at the end of the fiscal year in June 1917, the train was on the chopping block.[157]

It does not appear that Porter's successor, W. H. Cox, took the train out of storage after the passage of the summer. Instead, during this time, the Florida State Board of Health had its budget cut by 25 percent. As part of this process of reduction, "the health exhibit train was taken off the tracks."[158] In early January 1918, Cox attempted to sell the trains to the Illinois Department of Public Health. C. St. Clair Drake, the director, responded with regret that they would be unable to afford to such a purchase.[159] The state eventually sold the railcars to a carnival company.[160] Cox did not document what he did with the exhibits that were on board.

Appraising the Health Trains

For a brief period in the early twentieth century, state boards of health believed that health trains were a highly effective mechanism for spreading the gospel of health in urban and rural areas. Instead of transporting an exhibit to a limited number of locations that could accommodate large displays and an abundance of visitors and instead of spending time and money on installation and deinstallation, this new, purportedly cost-efficient, method brought the same exhibit to big cities and small towns. Officials took the lead in leveraging private and public partnerships to be able to create these mobile object-based public education projects. While official reports provided optimistic assessments of the train's appeal, evidence of its ability to effect specific significant change in individual sanitary practices remained elusive.

The history of California, Louisiana, and Florida's three health trains reveals health officials' struggles to actualize public health policies that encompassed preventive medicine. The health trains preached a gospel on the importance of constructing infrastructure and practicing personal hygiene to prevent the transmission of dangerous microbes. However, bringing examples of modernity that relied on electricity did not resonate with the reality of rural spaces, especially in the South, before mass infrastructure projects of the 1930s. While it seems certain that people turned out in high numbers to visit the train, health officials in California, Louisiana, and Florida were never able to pinpoint with any statistical certainty how that information changed actions and behaviors within localities.

While enthusiastically heralded at their inception, the health train was relatively short-lived educational movement. No state sustained a train as long as Louisiana's venture. Instead, state boards of health used them more typically as sporadic spectacles. In rural areas, especially the South, the trains brought a glimpse of modernity. However, politicians remained unconvinced of the train's utility, which in the end led to the demise of this experiment for popular public health education.

Chapter 4

Controversial Exhibits

Controversial exhibits exposed fault lines between and within communities. At times, they also created unlikely alliances. This chapter, which examines an exhibit about socioeconomic conditions in 1914 in Morristown, New Jersey, and a display about birth control in 1928 in New York City, demonstrates the fragility in the development of relationships that attempted to cross boundaries of class, gender, and ethnicity. Reformers interested in questions of public health found themselves at odds with each other and their constituents. Debates ensued over the utility and ethics of using exhibits as a form of popular education.

Scholarship on controversial exhibitions of culture, history, and health typically describes these types of episodes as late twentieth-century phenomena. Museums ran into conflicts as they began to mainstream social history into their displays.[1] The Bodies exhibits, which put plastinatized human cadavers in various states of dissection on display, have raised questions about the ethics of their production and the efficacy of using emotion for popular health education.[2] Studies of the arts, however, discuss in detail the uproar over the public display of visual representations of modernity in the early twentieth century, especially the Armory Show of 1913.[3] This chapter reveals that displaying modernity on other topics of the humanities, specifically interpretations of health and disease, also sometimes caused a public outcry in the early twentieth century. In the case of Morristown, Italian immigrants objected to reformers' descriptions of their family tableaus. In the case of birth control, there was disagreement about whether information about the human costs of reproduction could be discussed in the presence of children. While different content drove the particulars of debate, the failure of foresight to recognize the existence of significant cleavages between stakeholders remained a standard issue.

Controversy 1: 1914, Morristown, New Jersey

In 1914, Italian immigrants in Morristown, New Jersey, challenged the way in which an exhibit that was public health in nature characterized their homes as places in need of amelioration. They vehemently disagreed with captions that asserted that Italian bodies, especially of women and children, were the sites of cultural behaviors reformers needed to change. They tore the exhibit down from the walls. The incident both puzzled and served as a lesson for public health reformers. They both desired and resisted sharing authority and inquiry with their constituents.[4]

Reformers believed that they had identified spaces of poverty in need of repair. They based their conclusion on both a systematic study of the physical conditions and on their perception of the population that lived within. Reformers' desire to help did not disrupt their larger assumptions that immigrants from southern and eastern Europe were sources of disease.[5] How Italians viewed the construction of their neighborhoods and made health care choices was a different story.[6] The disconnect between the two groups fueled the controversy in Morristown.

Attracted by iron ore in the region, English colonists settled Morristown, New Jersey, in 1710. As the iron industry moved west in the nineteenth century and a rail link to Newark was established in 1838, the town's character changed. It became a residential suburb and home to some famous nineteenth-century cultural critics and writers, including Thomas Nast, Bret Harte, and Frank R. Stockton.

By the turn of the twentieth century, Morristown had grown into a relatively small urban municipality within the state. In 1910, the U.S. Census enumerated Morristown's population at 12,507, which was only a minor increase since 1900. The state assessed the town's infrastructure in 1915, a year after the controversy, and found it to be excellent: "There is a sewer system which drains all parts of the city, an abundant supply of pure water, electric and gas plants for lighting and power, a well-organized volunteer fire department equipped with auto apparatus."[7] Morristown appeared to be a livable city.

Morristown was home to a few small industries. According to the *Industrial Directory of New Jersey*, which the state produced to attract business and manufacturing, Morristown offered investors "a good supply of labor [that could be] obtained without difficulty."[8] In 1915, Common Sense Suspender Company was the largest employer in town. It employed forty people to produce suspenders and silk hosiery. Fourteen people found work at the John H. Schmidt Company, which made carriages and "auto bodies." Electric Alloy Company was the next biggest employer; twelve people worked there. Jas A. Muir, who made binder and leather boards, employed ten people.[9] These companies afforded working people—skilled and unskilled men and women—opportunities.

In the year after the exhibit debacle, some of Morristown's residents expressed ambivalence about expanding industrialization. The 1915 edition of the *Industrial Directory of New Jersey* noted some apprehension about the Morristown Civic Association's attempts to extend "inducements to attract industries to the city."[10] According to the directory, the association attempted to allay fears by arguing that it was looking to attract industries of the "right kind." Presumably, it was convincing because, by 1918, Morristown was home to two new woodworking companies that produced sashes, blinds, and doors and two new textile businesses that created muslin underwear and ladies' waists.[11] Between 1915 and 1918, the directory's calculation of the total numbers employed in local industries increased from 76 to 200 laborers.[12]

For those who worked in these enterprises, however, "wages, in many instances, [were] low and dictate[d] a standard of living for the home-town workers that contrast[ed] with the prosperity of the community residents."[13] Several oral histories of Italian residents remarked on aspects of the social geography of separation within the city. For instance, R. Sar Mischiara recalled working as a caddy over the summer as a boy at the Morris County Golf Club, and once the day's work was complete, he and his friends "got back to Flagler Street in a hurry . . . if we took too much time a policeman would tell us we were loitering."[14] Similarly, Luke Soranno remembered that the Italian groundkeeper for the golf club hired his mother and other women from the neighborhood to pull weeds to maintain the greens. The distance traveled between Flagler Street, which was the heart of the Italian community and the town's only dirt road in the early twentieth century, and the Morris County Golf Club was a tangible reminder of the disparity of wealth that existed in Morristown.

Even among the town's working community, there were divisions. Morris County hired some Italian masons to build its public library, St. Peter's Episcopal Church, and other structures befitting the county seat of government. Anthony Cherello recalled that these workers received more money for their labor and held themselves apart at Sunday morning gatherings.[15] The segmentation of labor extended beyond issues of skill. Rose Vigilante, for instance, remembered distinctions based on ethnicity. When she went to work in Morey LaRue's Laundry in 1910 at the age of thirteen, the Italian girls worked in the "basement, doing the flat work, folding pillow cases, handkerchiefs and sheets," while the "Irish girls worked upstairs on the street level, ironing the rich people's fancy clothes."[16] Charles Stelzle's 1914 assessment of the socioeconomic life of Morristown residents noted labor separation by race. He documented that young Italian women did not desire work as domestics. Instead, those jobs fell to African Americans.[17] Overall, class, ethnicity, and race played roles in shaping people's urban-labor experiences in Morristown in ways similar to other turn-of-the-twentieth-century cities.

The story of the destruction of the exhibit is part of a broader history of racial and ethnic tensions within the city. In 1910, the U.S. Census defined Morristown's population as 92 percent white.[18] The enumerators calculated that 8 percent of the population was African American (991 people).[19] The U.S. Census only classified nine residents in total as being "Indian, Chinese, and Japanese" in origin. Immigrants or persons with at least one parent who was foreign born constituted 47 percent of the town's white population. The largest immigrant population was Irish. The U.S. Census counted 894 people as Irish by birth and another 1,065 as having two parents who hailed from Ireland. Those with Italian heritage constituted the second-largest immigrant community in the town. The U.S. Census counted 798 people in Morristown as Italian and another 379 as having parents who were Italian. Nonetheless, in the eyes of the Bureau of Industrial Statistics of New Jersey, only Italians, Russian Jews, and Greeks constituted the "foreign immigrant element in the population."[20]

According to the Italian American Civic Society, Italians first came to Morristown in 1880 to help build the region's infrastructure. The Morris Aqueduct Company employed fifty laborers to help build a new reservoir. According to the society's memory, these workers did not receive a warm reception. As the workers made their way "through the town to their camp on Mendhum Avenue with their packs on their backs," they were greeted by a barrage of "angry comments over the foreign labor being brought" to Morristown.[21]

Twenty-seven years later, the organization celebrated its community's growth in population and economic prosperity. By its calculations, Italians owned a half a million dollars of real estate. The society argued that their affluence benefited the entire municipality. It cited the reduction of urban blight as evidence of the positive influence of Italians upon Morristown: "Flagler street which was the worst street in the town a few years ago, now has some of the finest buildings the town can boast of, concrete sidewalks, etc., and is populated exclusively by Italians."[22] The Italian American Civic Society was very mindful of public perceptions.

To the casual observer, however, there were distinct differences between the quarter square mile inhabited by this community and other parts of the town.

Despite improvements, much of the housing stock consisted of wooden apartment buildings. Outhouses were still the norm. The region was subject to flooding when the Whippany River overflowed its banks. Lastly, many of the residents, children included, earned a wage to contribute to family economies.[23]

In 1898, a group of people from the local Presbyterian church decided to create an organization (the Society for Work Among Italians) to administer social services for the Italian community in Morristown. Enoch Caskey spearheaded the endeavor out of a desire "to provide something for the Italian children whom she continually found in her backyard."[24] At first, the work consisted of offering access to domestic missionaries. The Society secured a room on Speedwell Avenue and retained an Italian student from Drew Seminary, Joseph Pasquali, to provide "Gospel Services" two evenings each week. The organization also directed him to spend one afternoon each week making house calls.[25] (Upon his death, Drew Seminary continued to send Italian students to work among the neighborhood's residents.) In addition to Pasquali, female members of the Society used the space to hold English classes for Italian men and a weekly sewing class for Italian women. When the building within which the room was rented burned to the ground in 1900, a community member gave the Society a new edifice on Flagler Street to house the "Italian Mission."[26]

In 1907, the Society for Work Among Italians decided to reorient its focus from religious work to "industrial and educational lines."[27] The Society created, in essence, a settlement house. Settlement houses were places where middle-class reformers provided a variety of social services and education programs in ethnic and minority communities that were designed to respond to the negative aspects of the modern industrial state. Hence, the Society's action was in keeping with similar creations across the nation.[28] However, this new emphasis met with resistance. In recounting her initial encounter with the community's residents, Marie A. Pierson remembered being met with hostility: "My little daughter was with me and several of the children in the neighborhood shouted 'Americana, Americana,' and began to stone her."[29] Although not as aggressive, the organization's monthly report from December 1907 noted that the children's behavior in Sunday school on December 15 was "very disorderly."[30]

Sometimes the Society's inability to exert control resulted in its use of police coercion to secure power over the community. While the group expressed regret over "feeling obliged to arrest three boys," it found that "the punishment seem[ed] to have had the desired effect."[31] The organization believed that as a result of its actions, "two of the boys arrested have been regularly to clubs with a marked improvement in deportment."[32] The settlement workers also felt that this action had "served as a check on older boys who have never come to the house but made a disturbance on the outside."[33] Once the Society learned to manipulate state mechanisms to secure compliance, which it interpreted as success, it decided to reformulate itself. In 1912, it permanently split its religious work and social work, and the renamed "Neighborhood House" became a secular settlement house. This action was not unique. Most settlement houses claimed to be nondenominational to allay any fears about trespassing against the intended audience's religious faith. Sometimes reformers actions, however, belied their preference for Protestantism.

Neighborhood House located itself in a two-story wooden structure at the top of Flagler Street. It had a gym, library, infirmary, several classrooms, a shower, and bathroom facilities. Although Catholic parents continued to find the Protestant proselytizing off-putting, many of the neighborhood children took advantage of the resources available.[34] The administrators of Neighborhood House expressed confidence in their public reports that they had established a relationship of mutual allegiance with the Italian community that they desired to serve. The controversy over the exhibit revealed to reformers that they had mistaken the degree to which the Italian community trusted any non-Italian-run civic organization to speak for them.

In 1913, at the behest of Morristown's local Protestant rectors and pastors, the Presbyterian Board of Home Missions (a national organization headquartered in New York City) conducted a six-month social survey of the city. The goal was to assess living conditions, housing, schools, and other aspects of life related to the health and well-being of residents.[35] In the published minutes of the organization, the Bureau of Social Services for the Board of Home Missions noted that this survey was one of two they conducted that year in New Jersey. (The other was of New Brunswick.) The organization argued that the "careful and painstaking study [of Morristown] was made based on a house to house canvass" for which they used seminary students from Drew University.[36] Presumably, this provided some continuity with Neighborhood House's previous efforts in providing social services. At the same time, only one of the 166 matriculated students that year was of Italian heritage, which may have contributed to miscommunications between the students and residents as to what purposes the documentation they gathered was to be used and interpreted.[37]

In addition to sending the students to circulate throughout parts of the town, G. B. St. John, the head of Surveys and Exhibits for the Board of Home Missions, sent questionnaires to various civic groups in Morristown for information. He asked these organizations about their history, size, accomplishments, and goals. At the end of the form, John asked for any photographs so that he might include them in the planned exhibit that was to accompany the published report of his findings.

Based on its survey, the Board of Home Missions wrote a fifty-six-page report titled "Report of the Social and Religious Survey of Morristown, New Jersey." While John participated in gathering information for the report, the principal author was Charles Stelzle, and in later descriptions, it was often referred to as the Stelzle report. The topics ranged from participation in church services to the number of people arrested for allegedly committing crimes of "social evil." While Stelzle found much about Morristown to be agreeable, his focus was not on the positive. Instead, his introduction suggested that while Morristown "cannot come under the classification of a great city with its stupendous problems, yet many of the problems of the city are here."[38] Stelzle identified issues of people and place in contributing to urban ills: "here are found the foreigners, here are the colored people, here are big tenements, here are found over-crowding and congestion, bad housing and bad sanitary conditions."[39] Perhaps anticipating doubt about his findings, Stelzle proclaimed that the study's "findings [were] not opinions nor hearsays, but facts."[40] Many in Morristown, however, contested his assertions.

Stelzle identified several specific issues he believed created a dangerous environment for the city's youth. According to his calculations, 12 percent of the children in Morristown attended school for only half the year because the town lacked enough space to accommodate them.[41] He asserted that the lack of access to full-time public education made for a dire situation. Outside of school, Stelzle believed that the city was delinquent in efforts to police public morals of popular amusements for its youth: "The state law forbidding children under 16 years of age to attend motion picture shows unless accompanied by an adult is constantly violated in Morristown."[42] While he noted the presence of organized sports, Stelzle found the small number of public playgrounds (two) unacceptable. He argued it was a civic responsibility to craft spaces of play for children.[43] Lastly, in studying the city's vital statistics, Stelzle expressed alarm over the rate of childhood mortality for those under five years of age. These dangers to childhood echoed the same types of perils reformers identified in other urban areas during this period. Nothing here was unique.

Stelzle's statistics that posited a relationship between seasonal labor and crime spoke to another reform trope. While he did not find that Morristown had more crime than other cities of its size, Stelzle believed that Morristown had enough issues to keep the police "busy."[44] Analyzing police records, Stelzle calculated that laborers committed the overwhelming number of criminal offenses

(49.5 percent). His tabulation suggested that "white" Americans accounted for the majority of crime in the town (57.8 percent). However, he singled out Italians (differentiating them from "white") and African Americans as threats to the public order. According to his calculations, Italians accounted for 11 percent of all crime in Morristown and African Americans 16 percent.[45] In his review of the police department's records, Stelzle tabulated that most arrests were for "disorderly conduct" and "drunk and disorderly" (73.1 percent combined), and that of those arrests, 49.5 percent were laborers. He then drew a connection between his two findings: "The large number of unoccupied men standing on the street corners, especially in the foreign district, is a constant menace to the city." His report insinuated that the absence of a will for temperance combined with the opportunity for idleness was a public health problem.

Stelzle came up with nineteen recommendations for Morristown. Foremost, he believed that while the foreign born of Morristown was "of a good type," they needed "direction in the care of their children" and instruction in English. He argued that their homes were "often insanitary [sic], sometimes through failure of public officials to do their duty, through negligence of the landlords, as well as through their own fault." He advised city leaders to secure a "group of volunteer workers among the foreign-speaking people, the negro population, and others who need help of various kinds" to work to develop "personal relationships" to effect change. He viewed this as more efficient and effective than organizational efforts of outsiders.

The second recommendation was for a public health nurse to work in the community. The third was to fix the problem of space in public schools. The fourth was to enforce garbage regulation. The fifth was for the city's wealthier residents to provide employment opportunities to address the issues he thought were the result of seasonal labor. The sixth and seventh recommendations were related to infrastructure and leisure (building a new library and a gymnasium for the exclusive use of young women). His eighth through sixteenth recommendations related to the role of the church in attending to residents' spiritual, recreational, and health needs. The seventeenth recommendation called for the city to increase its funding for the Morristown Central Bureau of Social Service. The last two recommendations suggested to civic, religious, and social organizations that they create permanent mechanisms for gathering and analyzing data related to the health and welfare of all residents.

Using this report, the Board of Home Missions created an exhibit out of 150 charts, maps, and photographs.[46] The organization placed the exhibit in a storefront at 41 South Street. (It did not document the exact date of the installation.) This site was on the main business thoroughfare of the city and was located slightly southwest of the First Presbyterian Church.[47] This placement suggests that middle-class white residents of Morristown, not its Italian working-class residents, were the target audience. The Presbyterian Board of Home Missions' annual review of its work contended that "thousands visited" the exhibit and that "mass meetings were held, where the findings were given and recommendations made." The organization did not mention the different controversies that ensued about the exhibit.[48] It did not comment that local businessmen held a meeting the day after Stelzle presented his findings to contest his deductions. It did not remark upon the Italian residents' visceral rejection of the display two days later.

Those who lived in Morristown and who read the local papers were well aware that many in the local community expressed reservations about the report and the exhibit. In the days before the Italians destroyed the exhibit, the two papers produced by Issac R. Pierson (*Jerseyman* published on Fridays and the *Morris County Chronicle* published weekly) and the *Daily Record* publicized the growing number of negative critiques. Several issues made the report contentious.

Stelzle's first presentation of the board's findings occurred at a "community mass meeting" hosted by the First Presbyterian Church on Sunday, March 8, 1914. According to the local papers, pastors from a variety of the city's religious institutions—Methodist, Presbyterian, Episcopal, and Baptist—were present. In addition to religious leaders, the *Morris County Chronicle* reported the presence of a diversity of parishioners. Morristown's pastors had suspended regular evening church services that night so that they too could attend Stelzle's talk.[49] Afterward, retorts to Stelzle quickly appeared.

First, city officials contested Stelzle's findings the next night at a businessmen's meeting held at the YMCA. Francis H. Glazebrook, the secretary of the town's board of health, and J. Burton Wiley, the town's school superintendent, offered statistics of their own to contradict Stelzle's findings.[50] The survey claimed that Morristown's death rate was 50 percent higher than New York City. However, the board of health was able to challenge that statement by showing that some invalids who came to use the town's two hospital facilities were nonresidents. Their deaths contributed to the mortality statistics but, the board of health argued, did not reflect the actual rate for the city.[51] Glazebrook estimated the death rate at 15 percent per thousand as opposed to Stelzle's assertion that it was 21 percent.[52] Stelzle, who attended the meeting, responded that he had excluded out-of-town persons in his statistical analysis. There appeared to be no resolution on the difference of their mathematical calculations.

Wiley contested Stelzle's analysis of school retention. Wiley was relatively new to Morristown. A graduate of Lafayette College, Wiley had worked as a high school teacher in Red Bank before becoming the superintendent of Morristown's public schools in 1912. (He would continue in that position until the late 1940s.[53]) When he did, he inherited a logistical problem: more children than space. In particular, an increasing number of students were taking advantage of the opportunity to obtain a high school education. Morristown was hesitant to build a new school or to structurally expand the existing Maple Avenue edifice.[54] While Wiley acknowledged the problem of school facilities, he argued that Stelzle's analysis was misleading because Stelzle compared the number of students enrolled in first and eighth grades for the current year. Wiley claimed that Stelzle should have based his report on the number of eighth graders who had enrolled in first grade eight years prior. Wiley asserted that if Stelzle had done that, then he would have known that school retention was not a significant issue.[55] In discussing death and school retention rates, the debates indicated how little consensus there was over best practices for statistical analysis.

The *Daily Record*'s account of what Wiley said at the YMCA meeting set the fuse on the powder keg for Morristown's Italians. The *Daily Record* reported Wiley as stating the following:

> Mr. Wiley declared that the folly of preparing all the children for the academic courses has been seen, and the eighth grade is now divided into three divisions, the academic, commercial, and industrial. The boy from Flagler street and the negro boy received different work and are treated different because they do not have the same culture and environment as the ordinary white boy.[56]

The quote suggested that Wiley discriminated. Based upon the *Daily Record*'s account, rumors spread that Wiley "widely advocated the segregation of Italian and negro children in the schools."[57] This rumor played an essential role in spurring Italians into action against the exhibit.

In 1881, the New Jersey state legislature passed a law prohibiting localities from forcibly separating children by race and nationality. This action resulted in the closure of Morristown's "colored school," which had opened in 1877.[58] Instead, the town's African American children began attending the Maple Avenue school.[59] However, the law did not forbid localities from offering separate facilities at the grammar school level. While the debates about school accommodations did not directly reference issues of race, it is reasonable to assume that questions about how to place children into new spaces raised the issue of segregation. A doctoral dissertation on the subject from the 1920s by Hannibal Gerald Duncan cited Morristown as an example of the perpetuation of racial separation.[60]

The morning after Wiley's talk, "a crowd of about 200 Italian parents of schoolchildren assembled in Flagler Street and marched in a body to the Maple Avenue School to demand satisfaction from Mr. Wiley."[61] Some newspapers estimated the crowd at 300, others at 400.[62] Wiley asked the crowd to send in a small delegation to discuss matters. With Louis Temallo acting as an interpreter, Wiley told the group of six men (Louis Marinaro, Eney Grupelli, Emillo Bozzi, Leo Maschiare, Fred Lucia, and Carmine Verilli) that the three divisions "were for the benefit of the pupils and open to all that the divisions had absolutely nothing to do with race."[63] As part of his process of amelioration, Wiley wrote a letter to the *Daily Record* wherein he argued that "some of the best students in the schools are Italian children."[64] As the small group met inside, a number of the crowd (the *Daily Record* estimated about twenty) grew tired of waiting and turned their attention to the exhibit.[65] (They had to walk around the corner and down about two blocks to reach the storefront.) What they found infuriated them, and they destroyed the exhibit.

Without archival evidence of the exhibit itself, the only means to extrapolate what the exhibition presented is to read in between the lines of reportage on the event. According to the *New York Times*, the Italian community objected to the "employment of themselves, their children, and their homes as 'horrible examples.'"[66] The *Bulletin of Photography* noted that the photographs all "depict[ed] scenes in the Italian settlement" and were designed to encourage the "remedying of tenement conditions."[67] Eventually, the police were called in to quell the disturbance.

Several papers made mention of the case of Pellegrino Venecio (also reported as Pelegrino Venitio and listed as Pellegrin Venezia in the U.S. Census). According to the U.S. Census manuscript for 1910, Venecio had migrated to the United States in 1897. He was twenty-seven at the time of the exhibit. He was married and had three children.[68] The city directory listed his occupation as "laborer."[69] The one person in charge at the exhibit and present at the time of the event, Merrill Morris, identified Venecio as the ringleader of the destruction.[70] According to Morris, Venecio destroyed a picture of his wife and baby that was captioned "The Foreign Born Must be Taught how to Care for their Children." The police arrested him and charged him with "malicious mischief."[71] The local judge set the bail at $200, which a fellow community member, Louis Marinaro, paid.[72]

In the days after the tear-down of the exhibit, the *Daily Record* reported that two other Italian men, Fred Lucia and Carmine Verilli, were contemplating taking legal action against the exhibit for including images of their families.[73] Fedele [Fred] Lucia, as the 1920 U.S. Federal Census listed him, was thirty-six in 1914.

He was married to Maria D. Lucia, and the two had five children. Also, Lucia's brother, Camillo, lived with them. The Morristown City directory for 1912/1913 listed Lucia's occupation as "laborer."[74] Corvine [Carmine] Verilli would have been thirty in 1914. (The U.S. Census listed him as Verillo, but the city directories listed his name as Verilli.) In 1910, the U.S. Federal Census listed him as living with his father, Leonard Verillo, along with his seven brothers and sisters and three additional boarders. Verilli was married and had a young daughter. The combined household was seventeen people.[75] The Verillis ran a bakery to support their extended family.[76] Lucia and Verillo had been present at the meeting with Wiley, where they complained to him about representations of their families in the exhibit. However, it does not appear that they left that meeting to participate in the exhibit's destruction.

In the days following the demolition of the exhibit, other Morristown residents continued to engage in a debate in the local paper about Stelzle's report. The editors of the *Morris County Chronicle* did not take a stand on whether Stelzle's figures were correct. However, they did agree with him that Morristown needed more school facilities.[77] Vincent Azzara, the court interpreter for Morris County, wrote a letter to the editor in which he argued that residents did not "need no social evil hunters" to "point out to us our shortcomings."[78] He believed that local organizations ought to resolve whatever issues confronted the town. Azzara also faulted the *Daily Record* for the destruction of the exhibit. He thought that if the paper had not misreported Wiley's comments about Italian and African American children, then his "countrymen" would not have reacted the way they did.[79]

The Morristown Business Men's Association adopted a resolution condemning the report and the exhibit.[80] This organization, which represented over 100 of Morristown's businessmen, objected to the publication of photos that took what they believed to be exceptions and render them as universal examples.[81] The organization also objected to the *Daily Record*'s publication of an advertisement for the exhibit. The announcement in the classified section of the *Daily Record* stated, "Lost A Dead Dog, A Valuable Theatrical Property of the Social Survey, Liberal Reward will be paid for its return to 41 South Street."[82] The businessmen argued, "The dog purported to have been lost appeared in a photograph shown in the social survey exhibit on South Street, which showed it lying upon a pile of rubbish in the rear of a public building."[83] They did not find this bait amusing.

In response to the negative publicity, the sponsors of the report used the local newspapers to try to mitigate the damage. They wrote a justification, which the *Morris County Chronicle* and the *Daily Record* published. As representatives of the various churches in Morristown, they explained to the public that they had asked the Board of Home Missions to conduct the survey with the best intentions in mind. The goal, they argued, was to "ascertain as accurately as possible the actual conditions existing in this town."[84] They believed that the result was a carefully crafted critique of social services in the city.

The damage to the exhibit was irreparable, and it closed a half-day early. In its seven days, according to those who put the exhibition together, the exhibit attracted approximately 2,000 visitors.[85] Usually, social reformers would have looked at those numbers and hailed them as a measurement of success. In this case, however, the exhibitors acknowledged that the more that people came to see the exhibit, the higher the sentiment against the survey grew.[86]

News of the visceral reaction to the exhibit spread throughout the United States.[87] Public opinion was often on the side of the Italians. The *New York Tribune*, which was no fan of progressive reform, argued that "no person is so poor or ignorant as to be without some sense of pride or independence." The newspaper reasoned that "they certainly cannot be expected to enjoy having [been] portrayed as 'horrible examples.'" At the same time, the *Tribune* did not contest the general point of the exhibit, which was that immigrants lived in substandard housing conditions. The *Tribune* argued that the poor "whom this form of social service is intended to help do not live in squalor because they like it, but because they cannot help it."[88]

Not everyone agreed with the characterizations of events. An anonymous letter from "a social worker in Morristown" to the editor of the *New York Times* argued that "it is bad enough that the Italians of the town should have misunderstood [the exhibit's] purport" but that this prestigious paper had as well. The problem, the social worker argued, lay in the conditions within which the poor lived. She or he was worried that some might not be willing to come to the aid of the poor because of these events. The goal of the exhibit, the social worker maintained, was to place "scorn" on the "community" that permits poverty to exist.[89]

The *Survey*, the most influential journal of social reform of the period, published a lengthy piece in response to the controversy. The editors felt it offered reformers a moment to reflect on their methods: "The incident has raised sharp questions as to exhibit functions and methods and goes to show that a specialized technique must be used in popular social propaganda."[90] The editors believed that the exhibit failed for purely managerial reasons. They continued to believe that "the exhibit is probably the best single medium for presenting the survey findings in attractive and convincing fashion to the community."[91]

The *Survey* blamed the Presbyterian Board of Home Missions for the controversy. In conducting the investigation, which according to the editors was made "at the instance [*sic*] of a small group of Morristown ministers," it "lack[ed] [any] organized body of local public opinion to back up the findings, favorable or unfavorable." The *Survey* printed statements contesting the report's death rate statistics and school attendance, which repeated Glazebrook and Wiley's assertions that cast doubt on Stelzle's findings. The editors of the *Survey* argued that these mistakes provided a potent argument for the professionalization of social work.

The final criticism that the editors of the *Survey* laid at the feet of the Presbyterian Board of Home Missions was the way in which the organization promoted the exhibit. The first problem, according to the *Survey*, was the use of the tagline, "What is the Matter with Morristown?" As the *Survey* noted, many in the community did not feel there was anything wrong with their town, whether those living in the "costly homes and beautiful estates," those who were steeped in promoting Morristown's business enterprises, or those living in the Italian neighborhood. More than that, the *Survey* argued the visual representations also had to be accurate. People gave their permission to be photographed, but they did not necessarily agree with the captions that characterized the content. Photographs did not speak for themselves, and the role of the text was crucial in translating the visual to public audiences.

The editors noted that this was not the first time New Jerseyans interested in public health reform had gone about the process in the wrong manner. They cited an example wherein the New Jersey State Board of Health created a stereopticon exhibit about tuberculosis. One image showed a family of thirteen living in small rooms, and it was intended to demonstrate what to avoid. Millard Knowlton, one of the state's inspectors, had secured permission to take a picture of the mother, who was home, and her eleven children in one room. When she saw the presentation, however, she thought Knowlton framed the picture as a "plea for relief" and she "resented" the implication that she sought public aid.[92] As the *Survey* suggested, "pride in having the whole family photographed is easily dissipated by a neighbor's careless or insinuating remark."[93] The "Morristown incident" served as a warning to social reformers that they needed to take particular care to cultivate a relationship with the communities they were attempting to work with to create a higher standard of living for all.

Issac R. Pierson, the editor of the local Morristown paper, the *Jerseyman*, also raised the question of moral principles. In his weekly editorial of March 20, he asked readers whether the exhibit had been a "violation of ethics."[94] He argued that the nature of exhibits related to health issues demanded privacy for individual identities. He contended that exhibit makers could have used the same kinds of techniques employed by medical journals, such as to obscure faces, to provide anonymity.[95]

In contrast to the Board of Home Missions' exhibit, a tuberculosis exhibit that the local and state board of health arranged to run in Morristown from March 16 to 20, just days after the other exhibit closed, did not raise alarms.[96] The tuberculosis exhibit was housed in two rooms in the Methodist church and included models, photographs, and movies.[97] Regarding public programming, Wiley permitted the schools to bring children during the day, and a slate of talks was scheduled for adults in the evening. Included among the speakers were Wiley and William Knowlton, whom the state board of health put in charge of directing tuberculosis work. According to the *Daily Record*, interest by Italians was high.[98] Organizers asked Azzara to translate Knowlton's talk.[99] According to the *Daily Record*, the exhibit was well received.[100]

The contrast in reception between the two exhibits demonstrated how different audiences expected public health exhibits to display information with and for their communities. The inclusion of Azzara as part of the tuberculosis exhibit validated the ability of Morristown's Italians to participate in conveying public health information. Italians had a voice. In the case of the survey, Italians believed that the exhibitors corrupted perceptions. They did not view their family structures as a public health threat and took offense at those who suggested otherwise. Their response to the exhibit served as a cautionary tale to public health exhibit makers.

Controversy 2: 1928, Parents' Exposition, New York City, Birth Control

The controversy at the Parents' Exposition in New York City in 1928 over exhibiting materials related to birth control for popular education also hinged on a set of cleavages within an imagined community.[101] In this case, the imagined community engaged in the question of child welfare. Should child welfare include discussions of birth control?

The 1920s was a period of transition. Reformers who had worked to create prenatal and postnatal public health services for mothers and their children found success in the passage of the Sheppard-Towner Maternity and Infant Protection Act of 1921. Margaret Sanger founded the American Birth Control League (ABCL) in 1921 to lobby politicians to rescind laws that deemed the dissemination of reproductive information through the mail as obscene and to provide educational materials on the societal benefits of preventing pregnancy.[102] More and more birth control clinics opened their doors to provide married women with information on reproductive health.[103] The use of mass media, especially radio and film, became increasingly critical for reshaping conversations about contraception from radical to respectable in the public sphere.[104] As the controversy about displaying materials related to birth control at the Parents' Exposition in 1928 showed, however, the question of who and how people should learn about controlling their reproduction remained thorny.

In 1928, the United Parents' Association of Greater New York Schools, in cooperation with the City of New York's Board of Education, sponsored a week-long exhibition (April 21 to April 29) at the Grand Central Palace. Their goal was to provide parents with expert advice on "the gamut of parental problems from spanking to spinach." The *New York Times* argued that this exhibition differed from its commercial counterparts in that it was "the first time in the city's history [that] the primary industry is having a showing." It was also larger than any commercial exhibit the city had seen.[105] *Hygeia*—a leading contemporary journal of individual and community health produced by the American Medical Association for the public—characterized it as a "novel event."[106]

Founded in the early 1920s, the United Parents' Association (UPA) of Greater New York Schools functioned as a coordinating body for the over one hundred local parents' associations throughout the city.[107] The city's superintendent viewed it as an advocacy organization to help promote "intelligent, long-sustained interest, [and] hearty co-operation" between parents and the school system. The Association desired to address educational policy questions at a systemwide level rather than participate in resolving "matters of purely local interest affecting any one school."[108] Within a few years, the organization's mission came to focus on "the profession of parenthood."[109] In 1926, Robert E. Simon, the organization's president, argued that that group was the "connecting link between the educator, the experimentors, the research organizations and the general public" interested in the question of "parental education."[110] The Association, hence, attempted to appear and act as a nonpartisan organization.

Seven years after the Association's founding, the Parents' Exposition of 1928 became its most significant undertaking. It began planning this event in the spring of 1927 with the intent to "dramatiz[e] . . . graphically the need for parent education and [to] stimulat[e] public interest in educational matters."[111] At first, some advocated that this be of a "commercial character," but the UPA dropped this idea in short order.[112]

Holding the exhibit in the Grand Central Palace turned this exposition into a significant event. The New York Central Railroad built the thirteen-story structure in 1911 as part of a larger complex to cover the railroad tracks on both sides of Lexington Avenue. (The structure occupied the entire block of Lexington

Avenue between 46th and 47th streets.) The bottom three floors served as exhibition space.[113] The Parents' Exposition used all of them. In preparation, the Exposition distributed almost three million tickets to parents and schoolchildren.[114] In the *New York Times*, the Association attempted to entice the public to attend with advertising that described the event as "stirring, colorful, and progressive."[115]

According to Roberta Christina Claus Ernst, the chairwoman of the Exposition committee, the purpose of the exhibit was to educate the community on all the "practical applications[s] of modern education."[116] The editors of the journal, the *Home Economist*, agreed. In notifying their audience of the upcoming event, they said, "Such an exposition marks a step forward in the modern educational effort that is being made to link more closely the theories taught in the classroom to community activities and to show the application of scientific truths to everyday practice."[117] The editors noted that the work of the "community's educational, social, civic and industrial experts" would be on display.[118]

As a further enticement, radio stations WGBS and WEAF began broadcasts about related topics three weeks before the Exposition began. These brief discussions offered the public a sense of the breadth of the exhibit. People could tune in to hear a session with the National Field Secretary of the Camp Fire Girls on "Ways of Making Your Daughter's Leisure Count." On a different day, parents could listen to a piece on "How to Simulate the Child's Interest in Art." The organizers consciously wanted to cross gender lines and, hence, advertised the exhibit with a piece titled "What a Father Finds Out about His Children When He Enters the Nursery."[119] During the exhibition, WGBS gave radio talks each day on a different feature.[120]

In speaking with a reporter for the *New York Times*, approximately eight weeks before the Exposition was set to open, Robert E. Simon, the president of the United Parents' Association, described the magnitude of the planning. He argued that "for the first time a graphic and unified picture of the whole subject of . . . child hygiene and parental education." The underlying argument Simon intended for visitors to take away was that "parenthood requires definite training and intelligent preparation."[121]

The exhibits covered a broad range of displays, which a diversity of organizations created. The Association divided the exhibition into four main sections: the home itself, the inner needs of the child, character education, and "the largest and most elaborate of all the divisions," which was devoted to education. Although the Association supervised the exhibit in its entirety, they left specific content up to a committee composed of ninety-three different educational experts.[122] These experts put people, pictures, and objects on display. The point,

according to William Hurk Kilpatrick, a professor of the philosophy of education at Teachers' College at Columbia University, was to explain the tenets of
"modern education" through observation. He believed that a child did not learn
unless he "sees the thing."[123] The same philosophy guided the exhibit.

For instance, the State Federation of Women's Clubs sponsored a display
to demonstrate the "esthetics [sic] of the living room." The goal, explained by
Mary H. Gregory, was to show how a "living room" could function as a "more
entertaining background for the social life of the family." However, Gregory was
not content to let the space remain static. Instead, "fourteen playlets, two a day
during the exposition week, show[ed] family social life at its constructive best."
This use of drama made the site come alive. Audiences watched as a family
"play[ed] games, entertain[ed] friends, danc[ed], s[ung], and play[ed] the piano."
Gregory desired to create "a living demonstration of how to be happy at home."
The living room functioned as a supervised site of leisure.[124]

On the second floor, Sidonie Gruenberg, the director of the Child Study
Association of America (CSA), was responsible for arranging the part of the
exhibit that focused on "Child Nature and Child Nurture." The United Parents'
Association believed that this would be "one of the most colorful spots of the
whole exposition." It was here that parents could find out about preschool education, for instance. Modeled after one used by the Teachers College of Columbia University, the CSA constructed a special sleeping room, playroom, kitchen,
and bathroom. Behind the display, they placed information about the major
objects of nursery schools. In this case, "stereopticon slides of babies at work
and play in such schools" served to heighten visitors' engagement with the
display.[125]

The third floor was, perhaps, the noisiest. The New York City Board of Education allowed 5,000 children to attend school at the exhibit.[126] These children
drew, modeled, recited, repaired automobiles, worked with sheet metal, and
made straw hats. In one corner, they also operated a printing press. Each day,
they produced a newspaper about the city's school system and printed 5,000
copies for distribution.[127] The UPA viewed the Board of Education's participation as crucial for the success of the event, a point that the Board of Education
also recognized. Consequently, the Board made it a "condition that all its
expenses should be met by the U.P.A."[128] The UPA fulfilled the request.

Writing a letter to the editor of the *New York Times*, Robert E. Simon, the
president of the United Parents' Association, encouraged the public to go see
this "most unusual opportunity . . . to see what is being done in our public
schools, with children demonstrating it." He argued that "it would take several

months to tour this city and visit all of the schools necessary in order to see the examples of all the work on exhibition."[129] Simon, as did the rest of the organizers, believed that the Exposition made ideas about education visible and tangible. Although it did not attract millions, the Association's final estimate was that over 250,000 persons visited the exhibit.[130]

Sex education was initially just one of many topics included at the exposition. As described to the public in the *New York Times*, "sex instruction" was a part of a section on "child nature and nurture." Gruenberg, who was in charge of the larger section, placed this topic together with questions of "obedience, punishment, health, food, recreation, play, religious education, and character training."[131] She involved experts on the subject. Dr. Harry Beal Torrey, of the American Social Hygiene Association and author of *Biology in the Elementary Schools and Its Contribution to Sex Education*, was on the planning committee for this section.[132] Also, Cecile Pilpel, a member of the Child Study Association of America and author of *When Children Ask about Babies*, was one of those listed to give talks.[133]

In December 1927, the United Parents' Association invited the American Birth Control League (ABCL) to participate, and in February, the ABCL signed a contract.[134] One can imagine the ABCL's surprise when, on the night of April 19 (two days before the exhibit was set to open), the president of the United Parents' Association, Robert E. Simon, informed the ABCL that he had to bar its participation. Harold G. Campbell, associate superintendent of schools, acting with the approval of Superintendent William J. O'Shea, threatened to withdraw the participation of the Board of Education if the Association did not ban the ABCL.[135]

The ABCL contended that nothing in its display was inappropriate.[136] The materials, including films, would present birth control as a topic of child welfare and public health. Campbell, however, believed that "as a matter between adults that's one thing," but the presence of children, he believed, changed the dynamic. He argued that if he did not take this measure, he would have "a thousand parents on my neck."[137] O'Shea argued that "we don't wish to have young boys and girls made acquainted with that sort of information, especially under school auspices."[138]

The ABCL countered in several different ways. First, it requested that O'Shea "appoint a committee to view the exhibit and 'suggest possible improvements.'"[139] The organization noted that it had taken part in similar events, including the Sesquicentennial Exposition and the annual Women's Arts and Industries Exhibition. In both cases, the ABCL claimed, its "exhibits have

received favorable comment from educators and scientists for their high standards and dignity."[140] When O'Shea denied the request, the ABCL remained
undaunted.

The organization rented space in a store (479 Lexington Avenue) directly
across from the main entrance to the Grand Central Palace. In the large glass
window, they placed a sign, "Forced out of the Parents' Exposition, the American Birth Control League Exhibit is Now Here-Come In." According to the *New
York Times*, the exhibit "drew crowds all day long."[141] Eleanor Dwight Jones,
the director of the exhibit booth, accompanied Margaret Sanger and Charlotte
Wyeth Delafield over to see Robert E. Simon, the president of the United Parents' Association, to ask him to place a sign up to explain why the ABCL's booth
was vacant and to direct people across the street. (The ABCL remained listed as
the exhibitor at booth "50-A" in the official program.[142]) The ABCL claimed that
if Simon honored its request, the ABCL "would accept the refund of its rent and
waive its rights under the contract signed by officials of the United Parents'
Associations."[143] Although Simon appeared agreeable, the newspaper reported
that O'Shea allegedly refused to allow the compromise. Jones argued "this [was]
tyranny."[144]

The ABCL used the public press to advocate for its position.[145] The organization gave the *New York Times* copies of two letters of support. The first was
from Kenneth Macgowan, who was a significant figure in the world of theater.
He had been asked to speak at the Parents' Exposition on "The Relations of the
Theater to Education and the Child." He sent a letter to Anne Lee, the educational director of the Exposition, and a copy to the ABCL. He argued that after
reading the newspaper reports about the banning of the ABCL, he could not
accept the invitation to speak. He argued, "Such self-appointed censorship by
any exhibitor or institution would be bad enough, but coming from the Board
of Education it is inexcusable."[146]

The second letter the ABCL made public came from Bruno Lasker, a relatively well-known writer and social worker. He had been invited by Evart G.
Routzahn of the Russell Sage Foundation to sit on a committee to "evaluate" the
exposition. Lasker declined to participate because he felt that "by its arbitrary
exclusion of one exhibitor at the behest of another the enterprise has forfeited all
claim to be taken seriously by educators as an impartial survey of educational
movements."[147] The *New York Times* printed these letters in full.

The press, however, sometimes used the controversy for its ends. *Time* magazine discussed the events as a means to criticize the entire endeavor. In a brief
editorial piece entitled "Parents," it claimed that "many people are parents" and
"many parents are stupid." Nothing that the editors saw at the Parents' Exposition

convinced them that it those parents would be better educated as a result of visiting the exhibition. Instead, the editors suggested that the entire endeavor "lacked" any "adequate demonstration of methods actually practiced by conscientious modern mother." While *Time* magazine did not take a position on the ABCL's display, its satirical criticism of the event itself lent legitimacy to the ABCL's claims against the organizers.[148]

According to the ABCL, the result of this publicity was not entirely negative. Jones suggested that "more persons had visited [the exhibit] than might have done so if the contract had been canceled." Nonetheless, she "resent[ed]" that O'Shea rejected the exhibit without actually viewing it.[149] Although Sanger felt vindicated by the press coverage, she argued, "No: we cannot claim a victory."[150] She viewed the controversy as part of a larger struggle over the censorship of information related to birth control. In particular, she regarded this event within two major political events of the time: a debate within the New York legislature that occurred a few months before the controversy and the upcoming presidential election within which a Catholic was running a serious campaign.

The debate over whether the New York legislature should adopt a law to allow physicians to provide birth control information to their married female patients was not new in 1928.[151] However, the types of support it got in 1928 were. The Women's City Club, which counted 2,500 members, had for a decade decided against supporting similar legislation.[152] After listening to two different physicians present on the pros and cons of the law, the club members voted via a secret referendum to endorse the legislation. It was not, however, an unqualified approval. The referendum stated that they would support revising the criminal code to allow physicians to advise married persons about birth control if the amendment received public backing "by recognized medical groups of high standing, such as the Academy of Medicine and the Committee on Maternal Health."[153] The referendum also made clear to club members that this endorsement would be from the Club and not imply any endorsement by single individuals.

Not all women's organizations approved. For instance, female members of the National Council of Catholic Women adopted a formal resolution to protest the legislation. They voted "to continue actively the protest against all legislative measures, whether in the nation or in the State, which would permit the dissemination of information resulting in birth control, and so undermining the sanctities of family life."[154]

Sanger decided that O'Shea's actions at the Parents' Exposition stemmed from his religious faith. She argued that his actions represented "a flagrant example of the tyrannical intolerance and usurpation of power exercised by office-holders born and bred in the Roman Catholic faith."[155] New York politics merged with presidential politics because the governor of the state, Alfred E. Smith, was running for president. Sanger asserted that the public should fear Smith's candidacy. O'Shea responded that "religion played no part in whatever action [he] took" to the exhibit.[156]

As proof of a Catholic conspiracy, the ABCL offered the example of Heywood Broun. Broun—a rather famous New York journalist—publicly objected to some of the reportage on the conflict. In particular, he spoke out against the "attitude" of his employer, the *New York World*, in an article in the *Nation*, for which he had a regular column. He wrote that the *World*'s editorial on the events in question displayed a "certain squeamishness" and as lacking in "courage." Broun believed the *World*'s editors had taken a stance against the ABCL's participation at the Exposition because they "live[d] in mortal terror of the power of" the Catholic Church.[157] In response to his post, the *World* fired Broun. The ABCL argued to their readers that although the *World* "claim[ed] to be more liberal than most of [the press] on the question" of birth control, "in regard to the tyranny of the Roman Catholic element," the paper's actions spoke otherwise.[158]

A few months after the Parents' Exposition and these debates about the politics of birth control, the ABCL had a booth at the Women's Activities Exhibit in New York in October 1928. This time there was no controversy. The ABCL noted that although there were some critics, most who stopped by the display "express[ed] approval." In addition to presenting printed material, the ABCL played a "silent lecture and moving picture." The ABCL found the public particularly engaged by this method of education: "This film was never without a crowd in front of it, some of whom were too shy to speak to the helpers in the booth, while others had their courage bolstered up by what they saw to the point of asking for more information." In this case, the organizers supported the ABCL's inclusion.[159]

However, the question of whether to provide public education to children about birth control as an aspect of social hygiene remained unresolved. Just a year after these events, the issue of birth control confronted the United Parents' Association once again. In June 1929, the UPA received word that Congressman Fiorello LaGuardia had introduced legislation to the House of Representatives to amend the federal obscenity law to allow information about sexuality to be distributed via the mail if it was medical or scientific and to be used for educational purposes.[160] The organization was informed that "all organizations interested in education" were asked to endorse the bill. Judging from the agendas and minutes of the UPA, this request posed quite a quandary. For the next six months, the organization debated the question of endorsement.

Initially, it looked as if the UPA would take swift action. In the minutes of the June 13th meeting, the UPA's governing board decided to send the bill in question to the board members who were not present at the meeting. The UPA also moved to take a position at its September meeting.[161] When the board returned to the question at its September meeting, however, it referred the matter to a newly formed subcommittee, the Law Committee.[162] The agendas for the UPA's October, November, and December meetings all listed an intention for Edgar M. Souza, chair of the Law Committee, to deliver a report on the question of "Endorsement by the U.P.A. of Bill to Amend Federal Obscenity Law."[163] The delay in action suggested an internal conflict.

The UPA came to a final resolution at its December meeting. It chose to avoid taking a position permanently. Although it did not make specific reference the bill, the UPA decided that "this organization should primarily interest itself only in such legislation as affects the children of the City of New York directly."[164] The UPA also declared that this position "should not be construed as limiting our interest in any vital subject affecting children, whether in the City or the nation, provided it is not a political question."[165] Taken together, the two sentences represent the unarticulated divisiveness that existed among the board's members. The UPA attempted to resolve this conflict by designating a process to facilitate civil conversation about controversial topics in the future. The UPA moved that the organization could take a position if "full information on the various sides of the question be secured before any action is taken, and ample notice be given to every member of the Governing Board prior to the meeting at which the question is to be discussed."[166] While nothing about this language adopted at the December meeting mentioned the federal obscenity bill, all discussion of that legislation ceased after this session.

The United Parents' Association held another Parents' Exposition in 1929, this time without any mention of birth control. The UPA installed a much stricter control over the exhibit process and focused on a central theme.[167] Over the next few years, however, the organization became ambivalent about the use of exhibition for popular education. In analyzing its exhibits, the UPA found that "deeper gains were difficult to discern." Once it examined the "cost in time and energy . . . it was decided not to make the exposition an annual feature of the [UPA's] program."[168] Overall, it decided that exhibits fell "short both of its purpose of raising money and as a means of dramatizing parent education."[169] While it did not mention the issue of birth control in abandoning exhibition, the steps the UPA took after its first foray into exhibit making indicated that it had not anticipated the types of problems that arose when attempting to craft a public health presentation for a mass audience.

Conclusion

In a time when exhibits were frequent, only a few issues seemed to arouse public controversy. When exhibits became personally offensive, they could be combustible. In the case of the Italian community of Morristown, it rejected the characterization of its families as a public health threat. The political and economic establishment in Morristown commiserated with the Italians' anger, since they too objected to the exhibit's negative depiction of the city. Although community insiders had initiated the study, outsiders produced the report and exhibit. As a result, the display did not comport with Morristownians' perceptions of themselves and their community.

In the case of birth control, the UPA needed the cooperation of the city's school system to ensure the success of its exhibit. In doing so, it sacrificed its relationship with the ABCL, even though the UPA viewed birth control as an aspect of child welfare. Those who came to the ABCL's defense did so because they viewed this as an act of censorship. Anti-Catholic sentiment also played a role.

Both controversies illuminated gaps between exhibit producers and consumers. Each interest group in these stories recognized the significance of visual representations, or they would not have felt the need to protest. The Italians were excluded from representing themselves. The ABCL was excluded from connecting with parents, especially those who might not want to have any more children. Despite the evidence of inflamed passions, neither reformers nor public health officials were permanently dissuaded from using exhibition for popular education. Moreover, audiences still attended.

A Gradual Decline

No single moment marked the death-knell for health exhibits as a tool for popular health education. Nonetheless, it is clear that by the mid-twentieth century, reformers and public health officials had gradually discarded the method. Reading the *Survey*, for instance, reveals that the number of articles and news briefings that discussed exhibits diminished significantly by the mid-1920s. At the same time as the decline of health exhibition, alternative mechanisms for mass communication appeared. Reformers and health officials took advantage of the advent of movies, the radio, and eventually television to connect with the masses.

While the impetus to routinize health exhibition as a mechanism of popular public health education dissipated, the notion that visuals could be used for health instruction persisted. Instead of temporary displays, however, the call came for permanent installations. Americans drew their inspiration from the Germans, whose Deutsches Hygiene Museum had been revamped in 1931. Speaking to his peers in public health in the United States, Homer N. Calver, director of publication of the Milbank Memorial Fund, expressed hope that a building could be found to house exhibits that "would visualize all health problems related to the more common diseases in a manner so graphic and dramatic as to command the attention of the average layman and be readily understood by him."[1] He called this strategy the "museum method" and argued that it was a "means of reaching thousands of individuals who are now indifferent to other appeals."[2] In 1939, Calver attempted to realize his goal at the New York World's Fair.

Officially titled the American Museum of Health (AMH), visitors to the New York World's Fair knew it as the "Hall of Man." The goal was to impart knowledge through these awe-inspiring visual engagements. A twenty-two-foot mural of a man with a glowing red heart greeted audiences, whose auditory senses were simultaneously stimulated by the background sound of a heart-beat. Visitors could peer into the human form in a variety of ways. For one, they could consider a transparent model of a man whose organs lighted up as a recording explained the corresponding physiology. After the fair's conclusion in 1940, the exhibit journeyed to several different locations, where it was put on temporary display. Organizers hoped to find it a permanent home but failed.[3] However, a few other health museums came into creation.

In 1940, the Cleveland Health Museum opened. Bruno Gebhard, one of the organizers of the Hall of Man, served as its director.[4] He argued that "health museums [were] science museums dedicated to the dissemination of information and education; their goal [was] 'To make Health Visible.'"[5] While these types of institutions did not exist to collect and preserve materials (the traditional conception of a museum's mission), he believed that these organizations embodied the ideas of "objectivity," "permanency," and "trust" that people associated with the term *museum*.[6]

In the twenty-five years between the Cleveland Health Museum's opening and Gebhard's review, very few other similar institutions were created. He counted six devoted to health, three devoted to medicine, and seven exhibits that were embedded in larger science museums.[7] Gebhard also acknowledged the limits of these museums. He noted, "We know very well that knowledge does not automatically change behavior."[8] Nonetheless, he still expressed faith in the power of visuals: "It is still true that seeing is believing—and in our field seeing is often relieving."[9]

Gebhard's continued faith in the value of the visual speaks to the optimism reformers and health officials possessed about the possibility of inspiring people through popular public health education. At the same time, the difficulties in sustaining museums of public health provided evidence again about the complicated nature of design and sustainability of exhibition as a mechanism for teaching the masses. As demonstrated throughout this text, exhibits were never that easy to create and maintain. It was also very unclear what visitors took away from their experiences. Did visual optics transform behavior? Did the exhibits transmit knowledge that empowered audiences in how public health officials and reformers intended? Those puzzles remained. Still, for a time in the early twentieth century, reformers and public health officials believed that exhibition was the most efficient and effective mechanism for instructing people, old and young, rural and urban, and black and white, in how to prevent the spread of contagious disease and create a stronger, healthier society.

Acknowledgments

Writing acknowledgements is a daunting task. I apologize now if I have forgotten to thank someone. Between directing an academic program, teaching, researching, writing, and parenting twins, I'm a bit forgetful at times. So, honestly, let me know if I forgot you and I will apologize with a frosty beverage of your choice.

Thank you to the many who have provided financial support for this project. My gratitude goes to Florida State University's Council on Research and Creativity for a Committee on Faculty Research Support award; to Florida State University's Dean of the College of Arts and Sciences, Sam Huckaba, for additional research support; to the Rockefeller Archive Center for a research grant; and to the New Jersey Historical Commission for a research grant. In addition, I thank the archivists at the Rockefeller Center Archive, the North Jersey History & Genealogy Center, the Louisiana State Archives, the New York Municipal Archives, and the State Library and State Archives of Florida for helping me to identify relevant material.

My thanks to Christian Juergens for translating Fraktur German for me. My thanks to Paul Pipik for the research help at the Michigan State Archives and Clarke Historical Library at Central Michigan University.

My thanks to Shauna Mulvihill for taking photographs for me at the California State Library.

I have presented versions of this material in a variety of formats. My thanks to the USC/Huntington Working Group in the History of Medicine and Public Health for their very constructive criticism on an early draft of the health trains chapter. (My many thanks to Carla Bittel for arranging that opportunity.) I have also benefited from constructive comments on these materials while presenting at the annual conferences of the American Association for the History of Medicine, the National Council on Public History, and the International Federation of Public History Annual Conference.

I am very grateful for the constructive criticism from Susan L. Smith and the anonymous reader of this manuscript. Their ideas on how to clarify and strengthen my arguments were exceptionally useful. I am also indebted to Peter Mickulas for his guidance on seeing this manuscript through from a draft to its final form.

I am grateful to my History Department colleagues, past and present, at Florida State. I'm especially thankful to Fritz Davis, Andrew Frank, and Suzy Sinke for their sage advice and willingness to always get a cup of coffee, find a seat on Landis Green, and chat about teaching, history, politics, children, pets, or a combination of all five.

Friends. They join you for food, drink, and fun. Sometimes they let you sleep in their extra bedrooms. They tell you not to give up when you get yet another rejection. Thank you to the late Michael Bottoms, Anastasia Christman, Susan Contente, Jane Dabel, Nathaniel Emerson, Ginny and Alexander Gulde, Lisa Materson, Heather McKay, Kurt Piehler, and Laura Talamante.

Family. Need I say more? I am beyond words grateful for my family's love and support. First, my mom, Susan Rosen. I love you. Your intellectual curiosity is contagious. Also, thank you for sending such beautiful photographs of the world. They put a smile on my face every time. A thank you to my stepdad Harold. Thank you to Ellen and Jeff Bontemps, Nick and Maureen Byrne, Kevin and Diana Byrne, Kelly and Frank McQuarrie, and the late John Byrne. Mary Byrne. I admire your strength, your kindness, and your down-to-earth advice. To the late Nicholas Byrne, I still seek your advice in spirit. Michael Koslow. Your sense of humor combined with knowledge of wine and theater makes every family gathering an event to remember. Carla Copeland, I admire your grace under pressure. Ulee and Ollie, you two make me laugh. Julian, big brother. Thank you for always being there when I need an ear and for always getting us a supply of fresh Fair Lawn bagels. Arnold. It is with great pleasure that I know your book will come out first. Your energy is infectious. I love you.

To my children, Benjamin and Ramona, Ramona and Benjamin. Every time I got frustrated with writing, you were there to take my mind in a different direction. I know I wasn't always grateful for the distraction, but in retrospect, I appreciated those breaks. You are my loves and I wouldn't have it any other way.

To Patrick. Another book. Another journey. Thank goodness you were able to find good music, good food, and good beer for us to share along the way or life at Constellation Court would be grim. Are you ready for another? Love you. Jen.

Notes

Introduction

1. Joseph Y. Porter Jr. to Joseph Y. Porter Sr., October 11, 1913, RG 894, Series 46, Box 44, Folder 19, State Archives of Florida, Tallahassee, Florida (hereinafter SAF). Key West was the fourth largest city in Florida in 1910 with 19,945 inhabitants. U.S. Bureau of the Census, *Thirteenth Census in the U.S. Taken in the Year 1910, Volume II: Reports of States, with Statistics for Counties, Cities and Other Civil Division* (Washington, D.C.: Government Printing Office, 1913), 298 and 331. I will discuss Porter Sr. in greater depth in Chapter 3.

2. U.S. Bureau of the Census, *Thirteenth Census in the U.S. Taken in the Year 1910, Volume II: Reports of States, with Statistics for Counties, Cities and Other Civil Division* (Washington, D.C.: Government Printing Office, 1913), 331.

3. I use the term *health reformer* to refer to those persons who engaged in public health reform whether or not they held a medical degree. On the professionalization of public health, see Elizabeth Fee, *Disease & Discovery: A History of the Johns Hopkins School of Hygiene and Public Health 1916–1939* (Baltimore: Johns Hopkins University Press, 1987). On the use of exhibits to communicate public health, see Julie K. Brown, *Health and Medicine on Display: International Expositions in the United States, 1876–1904* (Cambridge, MA: MIT Press, 2009). See also Nancy Tomes, *The Gospel of Germs: Men, Women, and the Microbe in American Life* (Cambridge, MA: Harvard University Press, 1998), 117–26; Lynne Curry, *Modern Mothers in the Heartland: Gender, Health, and Progress in Illinois, 1900–1930* (Columbus: Ohio State University Press, 1999), chap. 4; and Natalia Molina, "Illustrating Cultural Authority: Medicalized Representations of Mexican Communities in Early-Twentieth-Century Los Angeles," *Aztlán* 28, no. 1 (2003): 129–43. On the use of lantern slides as an instructional method for public health education in the interwar years, see Janet Golden, "The Iconography of Child Public Health: Between Medicine and Reform," in *Children's Health Issues in Historical Perspective*, ed. Cheryl Kranick Warsh and Veronica Strong-Boag (Waterloo, Ontario, Canada: Wilfrid Laurier University Press, 2005), 391–407.

4. Selling the importance of domestic hygiene for disease prevention to women occurred before the advent of the New Public Health, but the idea gained added urgency with the increasing recognition that microbes constituted the origin of disease. See Tomes, *The Gospel of Germs*, 62–67.

5. As Nancy Tomes discusses, immigrant women spent long hours attempting to maintain clean homes. Tomes, *The Gospel of Germs*, 190–92.

6. Marita Sturken and Lisa Cartwright, *Practices of Looking: An Introduction to Visual Culture* (Oxford: Oxford University Press, 2000), 168.

7. Brown, *Health and Medicine on Display*, 9; Tomes, *The Gospel of Germs*, 117–26.

8. Michael Sappol, *A Traffic of Dead Bodies: Anatomy and Embodied Social Identity in Nineteenth-Century America* (Princeton, NJ: Princeton University Press, 2002), especially chaps. 6 and 9; Carin Berkowitz, "The Beauty of Anatomy: Visual Displays and Surgical Education in Early-Nineteenth-Century London," *Bulletin of the History of Medicine* 85, no. 2 (2011): 248–78; Samuel J.M.M. Alberti, *Morbid Curiosities: Medical*

Museums in Nineteenth-Century Britain (Oxford: Oxford University Press, 2011), 21–22, 24, and chap. 6.

9. Bert Hansen, *Picturing Medical Progress from Pasteur to Polio: A History of Mass Media Images and Popular Attitudes in America* (New Brunswick, NJ: Rutgers University Press, 2009), especially chap. 4. On the use of photographs to prove bacteriological truths, see Jennifer Tucker, *Nature Exposed: Photography as Eyewitness in Victorian Science* (Baltimore: Johns Hopkins University Press, 2005), chap. 4.

10. Gregg Mitman, "Cinematic Nature: Hollywood Technology, Popular Culture, and the American Museum of Natural History," *Isis* 84, no. 4 (1993): 637–61.

11. Steven Conn, *Museums and American Intellectual Life, 1876–1926* (Chicago: University of Chicago Press, 2000), 4–5.

12. On the variety of visual ruses created for amusement in the nineteenth century, see James Cook, *The Arts of Deception* (Cambridge, MA: Harvard University Press, 2001).

13. Ibid., chap. 5.

14. Nancy J. Parezo and Don D. Fowler, *Anthropology Goes to the Fair: The 1904 Louisiana Purchase Exposition* (Lincoln: University of Nebraska Press, 2007).

15. The use of reenactors at living history museums continues to be an argument for their popularity. At times, however, questions about the historical accuracy of live performances raise debates about their ability to foster meaningful understandings of the past. See, for instance, Richard Handler and Eric Gable, *The New History in an Old Museum: Creating the Past at Colonial Williamsburg* (Durham, NC: Duke University Press, 1997); Richard Rabinowitz, *Curating America: Journeys through Storyscapes of the American Past* (Chapel Hill: University of North Carolina Press, 2016); and Amy Tyson, *The Wages of History: Emotional Labor on Public History's Front Lines* (Amherst: University of Massachusetts Press, 2013).

16. Karen A. Rader and Victoria E. M. Cain, *Life on Display: Revolutionizing U.S. Museums of Science & Natural History in the Twentieth Century* (Chicago: University of Chicago Press, 2014), especially chaps. 1 and 2.

17. Brown, *Health and Medicine on Display*, 1–10. Fairs were also understood to be respectable spaces in contrast to the allure of anatomy museums on the lower East Side of Manhattan designed to attract working-class men. See Sappol, *A Traffic of Dead Bodies*, 294–98.

18. Brown, *Health and Medicine on Display*, 196.

19. Each fair, with different degrees of effectiveness, provided emergency medical facilities for visitors and staff. Ibid., 194.

20. Julie K. Brown, "The Chicago Municipal Museum," *Museum History Journal* 3, no. 2 (July 2010): 231–56.

21. Julie K. Brown, "Connecting Health and Natural History: A Failed Initiative at the American Museum of Natural History, 1909–1922," *American Journal of Public Health* 104, no. 10 (October 2014): 1877–88. The 1911 International Hygiene Exhibition in Dresden also influenced Charles Edward Winslow, the department's curator. I will discuss this exhibit further in Chapter 3.

22. The Chicago Municipal Museum lasted two years. The Department of Public Health at the American Natural History Museum lasted thirteen years. Other attempts at health museums met with varying success in the twentieth century. See Elena Canadelli, "'Scientific Peep Show': The Human Body in Contemporary Science Museums," *Nuncius* 26, no. 1 (2011): 159–84; Erin McLeary and Elizabeth Toon, "Here Man Learns about Himself," *American Journal of Public Health* 102, no. 7

(July 2012): e27–e36; and Klaus Vogel, "The Transparent Man-Some Comments on the History of a Symbol," in *Manifesting Medicine: Bodies and Machines*, ed. Robert Bud, Bernard Finn, and Helmuth Trischler (Amsterdam: Harwood Academic, 1999), 31–61.

23. Kathryn H. Fuller, *At the Picture Show: Small-Town Audiences and the Creation of Movie Fan Culture* (Washington, D.C.: Smithsonian Institution Press, 1996), 7 and 17.

24. Ibid., 81.

25. Martin S. Pernick, "More Than Illustrations: Early Twentieth-Century Health Films as Contributors to the Histories of Medicine and of Motion Pictures," in *Medicine's Moving Pictures: Medicine, Health, and Bodies in American Film and Television*, ed. Leslie J. Reagan, Nancy Tomes, and Paula A. Treichler (Rochester, NY: University of Rochester Press, 2007), 19.

26. Ibid., 19–20.

27. Ibid., 31.

28. Martin S. Pernick, *The Black Stork: Eugenics and the Death of 'Defective' Babies in American Medicine and Motion Pictures since 1915* (Oxford: Oxford University Press, 1996), 148.

29. The literature on the use of film and television to communicate medical knowledge and norms in the twentieth century is considerable. Works that have helped to inform this work besides *Medicine's Moving Pictures* include John C. Burnham, *How Superstition Won and Science Lost: Popularizing Science and Health in the United States* (New Brunswick, NJ: Rutgers University Press, 1998); Lisa Cartwright, *Screening the Body: Tracing Medicine's Visual Culture* (Minneapolis: University of Minnesota Press, 1995); and Lester D. Friedman, ed., *Cultural Sutures: Medicine and Media* (Durham, NC: Duke University Press, 2004).

30. Fuller, *At the Picture Show*, 29–34.

31. Mitman, "Cinematic Nature," 653.

32. Curry, *Modern Mothers in the Heartland*, 91–98; Natalia Molina, "Illustrating Cultural Authority," 129–43.

33. Tomes, *The Gospel of Germs*, 117; Roland Marchand, *Advertising the American Dream: Making Way for Modernity, 1920–1940* (Berkeley: University of California Press, 1985), 154.

34. Homer N. Calver, "Marketing Mass Education," *American Journal of Public Health* 22, no. 1 (January 1932): 55. On the effective showmanship of the purveyors of patent medicine, see James Harvey Young, *The Toadstool Millionaires: A Social History of Patent Medicine before Federal Regulation* (Princeton, NJ: Princeton University Press, 1961), chaps. 8 and 12.

35. McLeary and Toon, "Here Man Learns about Himself," e31–e34.

36. Burnham, *How Superstition Won and Science Lost*, 3–4.

37. Ibid., 62.

38. Ibid., 38.

39. Ibid., 75.

40. Richard A. Meckel, *Classrooms and Clinics: Urban Schools and the Protection and Promotion of Child Health* (New Brunswick, NJ: Rutgers University Press, 2013), especially chap. 5.

41. George E. Hein, *Progressive Museum Practice: John Dewey and Democracy* (Walnut Creek: Left Coast Press 2012), chap. 2.

42. Ibid., chap. 4.

43. John Ettling, *The Germ of Laziness: Rockefeller Philanthropy and Public Health in the New South* (Cambridge, MA: Harvard University Press, 1981), 157–65.

44. William A. Link, "'The Harvest Is Ripe, but the Laborers Are Few': The Hookworm Crusade in North Carolina, 1909–1915," *North Carolina Historical Review* 67, no. 1 (January 1990): 15.

45. John Duffy, *The Sanitarians: A History of American Public Health* (Urbana: University of Illinois Press, 1990), chap. 14.

1. Developing Exhibition as a Common Tool for Popular Education

1. Kenneth D. Widdemer and Harry L. Hopkins, "Health Shop," *Hygeia* 9, no. 8 (August 1931): 740–42. Kenneth D. Widdemer, *A Decade of District Health Center Pioneering* (New York: East Harlem Health Center, 1932), map of East Harlem.

2. On the power and logic of maternalist arguments for bettering working, environmental, and social conditions, see Kathryn Kish Sklar, *Florence Kelley and the Nation's Work: The Rise of Women's Political Culture, 1830–1900* (New Haven, CT: Yale University Press, 1995). On the complexities of pursuing a maternalist strategy for reform instead of a feminist one, see Robert Johnston, *The Radical Middle Class: Populist Democracy and the Question of Capitalism in Progressive Era Portland, Oregon* (Princeton, NJ: Princeton University Press, 2003), chap. 2.

3. For examples, see "exhibits," *Survey* 29, no. 20 (February 15, 1913): 667; *Survey* 31 (March 21, 1914): 790.

4. Richard Harrison Shryock, *National Tuberculosis Association 1904–1954: A Study of the Voluntary Health Movement in the United States* (New York: National Tuberculosis Association, 1957), 62.

5. Ibid., 63. Pneumonia supplanted tuberculosis as the leading cause of mortality during this period.

6. Ibid., 28.

7. While the literature on the history of tuberculosis as experienced, regulated, and cured is vast, my work has been informed in particular by Emily K. Abel, *Tuberculosis & The Politics of Exclusion: A History of Public Health & Migration to Los Angeles* (New Brunswick, NJ: Rutgers University Press, 2007); Barbara Bates, *Bargaining for Life: A Social History of Tuberculosis, 1876–1938* (Philadelphia: University of Pennsylvania Press, 1992); Cynthia Connolly, *Saving Sickly Children: The Tuberculosis Preventorium in American Life, 1909–1970* (New Brunswick, NJ: Rutgers University Press, 2008); Tanya Hart, *Health in the City: Race, Poverty, and the Negotiation of Women's Health in New York City, 1915–1930* (New York: New York University Press, 2015); and Katherine Ott, *Fevered Lives: Tuberculosis in American Culture since 1870* (Cambridge, MA: Harvard University Press, 1996).

8. Robert Wiebe, *The Search for Order, 1877–1920* (New York: Hill and Wang, 1966).

9. "The American Tuberculosis Exhibition," *Charities and The Commons* 15, no. 4 (October 28, 1905): 121. Frank Dekker Watson, *The Charity Organization Movement in the United States: A Study in American Philanthropy* (New York: Macmillan, 1922), 294. The NASPT formed in 1904. New York's CSO formed in 1882.

10. Four years later, the American Museum of Natural History incorporated public health into its curatorial structure. Julie K. Brown discusses the 1905 exhibit as an antecedent to that step. See Julie K. Brown, "Connecting Health and Natural History: A Failed Initiative at the American Museum of Natural History, 1909–1922," *American Journal of Public Health* 104, no. 10 (October 2014): 1879.

11. Shryock, *National Tuberculosis Association 1904–1954*, 76.

12. Watson, *The Charity Organization Movement*, 295.

13. "For a Permanent Tuberculosis Exhibit," *Charities and The Commons* 15, no. 9 (December 2, 1905): 278.

14. Ibid., 278–79.

15. "Thousands at the Tuberculosis Exposition," *Charities and The Commons* 15, no. 10, (December 9, 1905): 345.

16. According to Julie Brown, the first major successful tuberculosis exhibit occurred in Maryland in January 1904. The first exhibit on tuberculosis at an international event happened that same year at the St. Louis World's Fair, but it was less successful. See Brown, *Health and Medicine on Display*, 177–78.

17. "For a Permanent Tuberculosis Exhibit," *Charities and The Commons* 15, no. 9 (December 2, 1905): 279.

18. "Tuberculosis Exhibition in Mexico," *Charities and The Commons* 17 (n.d.): 664; "Tuberculosis Exhibit in Toronto," *Charities and The Commons* 16, no. 24 (September 15, 1906): 595. In Mexico, the exhibit was displayed in conjunction with the annual meeting of the American Public Health Association. In Canada, it was shown in combination with the annual gathering of the British Medical Association.

19. "The Travelling Tuberculosis Exhibition," *Charities and The Commons* 16, no. 12 (June 23, 1906): 377.

20. Shyrock, *National Tuberculosis Association 1904–1954*, 101. Olivia Sage established the Russell Sage Foundation in 1906. For more on how Olivia Sage transformed her fortune into an important instrument for supporting social reform and antipoverty efforts, see Ruth Crocker, *Mrs. Russell Sage: Women's Activism and Philanthropy in Gilded Age and Progressive Era America* (Bloomington: Indiana University Press, 2006).

21. H.R.M. Landis, "The Tuberculosis Exhibition in Philadelphia," *Charities and The Commons* 15, no. 21 (February 24, 1906): 726. Landis was a physician working in Philadelphia.

22. Ibid.

23. Ibid.

24. "The Milwaukee Exhibition," *Charities and The Commons* 16, no. 12 (June 23, 1906): 378.

25. "Tuberculosis Exhibition in Chicago," *Charities and The Commons* 16, no. 2 (April 14, 1906): 91.

26. Ibid.

27. "The American Tuberculosis Exhibition at Manistee," *Charities and The Commons* 16, no. 23, (September 8, 1906): 587.

28. Mainstee's population was between 12,381 (1910) and 14,260 (1900). See report for Michigan, Table 1. Population of Minor Civil Divisions, 1910, 1900, and 1890. U.S. Bureau of the Census, *Thirteenth Census of the United States Taken in the Year 1910*, Volume II: Population, https://www2.census.gov/library/publications/decennial/1910/volume-2/volume-2-p8.pdf. I used 13,000 as a rough estimate in determining the percentage of people who visited the exhibit.

29. Gaylord S. White, "With the Traveling Tuberculosis Exhibition," *Charities and The Commons* 16, no. 12 (June 23, 1906): 382. Settlement houses were places where middle-class reformers provided a variety of social services and education programs in ethnic and minority communities that were designed to respond to the negative aspects of the modern industrial state. On the history of the settlement house movement in various forms, including religious, see Ruth Crocker, *Social Work and*

Social Order: The Settlement Movement in Two Industrial Cities, 1889–1930 (Urbana: University of Illinois Press, 1992); Allen F. Davis, *Spearheads for Reform: The Social Settlements and the Progressive Movement, 1890–1914* (New York: Oxford University Press, 1967); Maureen Flanagan, *Seeing with Their Hearts: Chicago Women and the Vision of the Good City, 1871–1933* (Princeton, NJ: Princeton University Press, 2002); Deirdre Moloney, *American Catholic Lay Groups and Transatlantic Social Reform in the Progressive Era* (Chapel Hill: University of North Carolina Press, 2002); and Robyn Muncy, *Creating a Female Dominion in American Reform, 1890–1935* (New York: Oxford University Press, 1994).

30. "The Travelling Tuberculosis Exhibition," *Charities and The Commons* 16, no. 12 (June 23, 1906): 377.

31. Ibid.

32. "Exhibits in Minneapolis," *Charities and The Commons* 21 (March 20, 1909): 1243.

33. Gaylord S. White, "With the Traveling Tuberculosis Exhibition," *Charities and The Commons* 16, no. 12 (June 23, 1906): 384.

34. Ibid., 386.

35. Ibid., 387.

36. Ibid.

37. "The Travelling Tuberculosis Exhibition," *Charities and The Commons* 16, no. 12 (June 23, 1906): 377.

38. "Tuberculosis Exhibit in Brooklyn," *Charities and The Commons* 17 (November 17, 1907): 325.

39. "Traveling Tuberculosis Exhibit, Maryland," *Charities and The Commons* 18 (July 20, 1907): 444.

40. "Tuberculosis Exhibit in Syracuse," *Charities and The Commons* 17 (November 17, 1907): 324.

41. Lillian Brandt, "The Keynote of the Congress," *Charities and The Commons* 21 (November 7, 1908): 185.

42. Lavery served as the president of the Milk Reform Committee in New York and was a friend of Theodore Roosevelt's. See Lavery's obituary in the *Indiana Gazette*, December 7, 1944.

43. James F. Lavery, "The Exhibit," *Charities and The Commons* 21 (November 7, 1908): 204.

44. Ibid.

45. Ibid.

46. "Chapter LXXV: Alfred Meyer, M.D.," in Adolphus Knopf, *A History of the National Tuberculosis Association, National Tuberculosis Association* (Philadelphia: National Tuberculosis Association, 1922), 461–62, https://books.google.com/books ?id=eyNAAAAAYAAJ&lpg=PA462&dq=alfred%20meyer%20tuberculosis&pg =PA461#v=onepage&q=alfred%20meyer%20tuberculosis&f=false.

47. "Tuberculosis Exhibit to Go to New York," *Charities and The Commons* 21 (October 17, 1908): 100; "The Exhibit as Measured by Carloads," *Charities and The Commons* 21 (November 7, 1908): 172.

48. "Tuberculosis Exhibit to Go to New York," *Charities and The Commons* 21 (October 17, 1908): 100.

49. Ibid.

50. Ibid.

51. Arthur P. Kellog, "Printer's Ink as a Preventive Agent," *Charities and The Commons* 21, no. 10 (December 5, 1908): 359–60.

52. "Tuberculosis Exhibit in New York," *Charities and The Commons* 21, no. 10 (December 5, 1908): 355.

53. "The International Tuberculosis Exhibition," *Charities and The Commons* 21, no. 11 (December 12, 1908): 411.

54. "Philadelphia's Exhibit," *Charities and The Commons* 21 (February 20, 1909): 1005.

55. E. G. Routzahn, "The Value of the Tuberculosis Exhibition," *Survey* 23 (November 20, 1909): 254. I will discuss Routzahn in greater depth in Chapter 2.

56. Ibid.

57. Ibid., 253.

58. Ibid.

59. Ibid.

60. Ibid.

61. Maureen Flanagan, "The City Profitable, the City Livable: Environmental Policy, Gender, and Power in Chicago in the 1910s," *Journal of Urban History* 22, no. 2 (January 1996): 163–90.

62. Lenora Austin Hamlin, "The Municipal Museum of Chicago," *Charities and The Commons* 15, no. 5 (n.d.): 171.

63. Julie Brown analyzes the museum's history within the context of turn-of-the-century reform movements and the history of museums. See Julie K. Brown, "The Chicago Municipal Display, 1904–1907," *Museum History Journal* 3, no. 2 (July 1910): 231–56. For more on Jane Addams, see Jean Bethke Elshtain, *Jane Addams and the Dream of American Democracy* (New York: Basic Books, 2001).

64. Hamlin, "The Municipal Museum of Chicago," 176. Daughter of a former governor of Minnesota, Lenora Austin married Conde Hamlin, the managing editor of the St. Paul *Pioneer Press* in 1892. Lenora was a major participant in women's club work in St. Paul and traveled to St. Louis in the spring of 1904 to manage the city's municipal exhibit at the world's fair. In response to her activities, Conde Hamlin sued for divorce on the grounds of desertion. Afterward, she moved to Jane Addams's Hull House in Chicago, where she became the director of the Municipal Museum of Chicago. Upon her divorce, Lenora traveled in Europe before eventually returning to St. Paul, where she continued to engage in reform activities. "Matrimony Notice," *Daily Inter Ocean*, December 11, 1892; "Club Work Is Divorce Cause," *Duluth News Tribune*, February 26, 1905; *Saint Paul Institute Bulletin* (December 1910): 3, https://hdl.handle.net/2027/nyp.33433012589929.

65. *Hull House Year Book* (1906–1907), https://archive.org/details/hullhouseyearboo 1906hull/page/52.

66. "Exhibit of Congestion," *Charities and The Commons* 19 (January 18, 1908): 1399.

67. "Opening New York's Congestion Exhibit," *Charities and The Commons* 19 (March 14, 1908): 1729.

68. John Martin, "The Exhibit of Congestion Interpreted," *Charities and The Commons* 10 (April 4, 1908): 27.

69. "New York's Problem of Congestion," *Springfield Republican*, February 19, 1908; Gregory F. Gilmartin, *Shaping the City: New York and the Municipal Art Society* (New York: Clarkson Potter, 1995).

70. Charles Mulford Robinson, "The City Plan Exhibition," *Survey* 22 (May 29, 1909): 314.

71. Ibid.

72. The *Charities and The Commons* had devoted an entire issue to the Pittsburgh Survey in January 1909. See *Charities and The Commons* 21, no. 14 (January 2, 1909).

Funded by the Russell Sage Foundation, the Pittsburgh Survey was instrumental in legitimizing sociological studies to prove problems of poverty existed and justified efforts for reform.

73. Robinson, "The City Plan Exhibition," 316.

74. Ibid.

75. On the shifting nature of municipal government, see Eric Monkkonen, *America Becomes Urban: The Development of U.S. Cities & Towns, 1780–1980* (Berkeley: University of California Press, 1988).

76. Letter to the Editor by R. C. Sanger of Franklin, N.H., *Survey* 25 (February 25, 1911): 886. New York appears to have held one in 1910, but the *Survey* did not report on it. It did, however, report on the second Budget Exhibit held in New York in 1911. "Second Budget Exhibit in N.Y.," *Survey* 26 (September 30, 1911): 899.

77. "Budget Exhibit in Two Cities," *Survey* 20 (April 22, 1911): 135.

78. Ibid., 136.

79. "Second Budget Exhibit in N.Y.," *Survey* 26 (September 30, 1911): 899.

80. "Milwaukee's Open Book," *Survey* 27, no 14 (January 6, 1912): 1443.

81. Ibid., 1444.

82. "Pittsburgh's Smoke Abatement Exhibit," *Survey* 31, no. 1 (October 4, 1913): 1.

83. "The Movement for Industrial Exhibitions," *Charities and The Commons* 17 (n.d.): 106.

84. "Exhibition of Safety and Industrial Hygiene," *Charities and The Commons* (July 7, 1906): 403.

85. *Social Progress: A Year Book and Encyclopedia of Economic, Industrial, and Social, and Religious Statistics* (New York: Baker and Taylor Company, 1904), 253, https://hdl.handle.net/2027/mdp.39015057286810.

86. Ibid., 403.

87. Ibid.

88. Joshiah Strong, "Museums of Security," *Charities and The Commons* 17 (n.d.): 814.

89. Mabel Hay Barrows Mussey, "Holding the Mirror Up to Industry, The Philadelphia Exhibit," *Charities and The Commons* 17 (n.d.): 592.

90. Ibid.

91. Ibid.

92. Ibid., 593.

93. "Philadelphia Industrial Exhibition," *Charities and The Commons* 17 (n.d.): 436.

94. Kate Sampsell Willmann, "Lewis Hine, Ellis Island, and Pragmatism: Photographs as Lived Experience," *Journal of the Gilded Age and Progressive Era* 7, no. 2 (April 2008): 221–52, especially 240–43.

95. "Chicago Industrial Exhibit," *Charities and The Commons* 17 (n.d.): 1078; Graham Romeyn Taylor, "The Chicago Industrial Exhibit," *Charities and The Commons* 18 (n.d.): 39.

96. "Chicago Industrial Exhibit," *Charities and The Commons* 17 (n.d.): 1028.

97. Taylor, "The Chicago Industrial Exhibit," 39.

98. Ibid., 41.

99. Brown, "The Chicago Municipal Museum," *Museum History Journal* 3, no. 2 (2010): 253.

100. Taylor, "The Chicago Industrial Exhibit," 39.

101. Ibid., 40.

102. "Massachusetts Industrial Exhibit," *Charities and The Commons* 18 (n.d.): 7.

103. Edward T. Hartman, "Boston's Industrial Exhibit," *Charities and Commons* 18 (n.d.): 144.

104. Ibid., 147.

105. Walter I. Trattner, "The First Federal Child Labor Law (1916)," *Social Science Quarterly* 50, no. 3 (1969): 511.

106. "A New Exhibit of Home Work," *Survey* 28, no. 1 (April 6, 1912): 8.

107. Ibid., 9.

108. Ibid., 10.

109. For more on this movement, see, for instance, Robyn Muncy, *Creating a Female Dominion in American Reform, 1890–1935* (Oxford: Oxford University Press, 1991); Molly Ladd-Taylor, *Mother-Work: Women, Child Welfare, and the State, 1890–1930* (Urbana: University of Illinois Press, 1994).

110. "The Child Welfare Exhibit Next Fall," *Survey* 24 (July 23, 1910): 615.

111. "Opening the Chicago Child Welfare Exhibit," *Survey* 26 (May 20, 1911): 282.

112. Maureen Flanagan, *Seeing with Their Hearts: Chicago Women and the Vision of the Good City, 1871–1933* (Princeton, NJ: Princeton University Press, 2002); Daphne Spain, *How Women Saved the City* (Minneapolis: University of Minnesota Press, 2001).

113. "Opening the Chicago Child Welfare Exhibit," *Survey* 26 (May 20, 1911): 282.

114. Ibid.

115. Ibid.

116. Sherman C. Kincsley, "Child Welfare—The Next Step," *Survey* 26 (June 10, 1911): 415.

117. I. K. Friedman, "Chicago Child Welfare Exhibit-Impressions," *Survey* 26 (June 10, 1911): 411.

118. Ibid., 410.

119. Ibid., 411.

120. "Opening the Chicago Child Welfare Exhibit," *Survey* 26 (May 20, 1911): 283.

121. Ibid.

122. "Child Welfare Exhibit in French and English," *Survey* 26 (July 22, 1911): 595.

123. "The Spirit of Youth and Kansas City," *Survey* 27 (December 2, 1911): 1272.

124. L. A. Halbert, "History of the Board of Public Welfare of Kansas City, Missouri," *Public Welfare* 1, no. 2 (May 1918): 19, https://hdl.handle.net/2027/uiug.30112046472509.

125. "The Spirit of Youth and Kansas City," *Survey* 27 (December 2, 1911): 1273.

126. Ibid., 1272.

127. Ibid.

128. "Travelling Exhibit for City Welfare," *Survey* 28, no. 1 (April 6, 1912): 6.

129. Ibid., 7.

130. "Through a Child's Eyes: What School Children Saw in a Child Welfare Exhibit," *Lexington Herald*, September 14, 1913; May Ayres, "The Child Welfare Exhibit through the Children's Eyes," *Survey* 30, no. 24 (September 13, 1913): 711.

131. Unfortunately, Aryes was not very specific in explaining the impetus for the survey. Using passive voice, she wrote, "The following week those in the upper grades were asked to write letters telling about what they remembered. Some 553 of these letters were examined."

132. Ayres, "The Child Welfare Exhibit," 711.

133. Ibid., 712.

134. Ibid., 713.

135. Ibid.

136. Ibid., 714.

137. "Child Welfare Exhibits to Fit Every Need and State," *Survey* 31, no. 5 (November 1, 1913): 106.

138. Ibid.

2. The Art of Exhibit Making

1. Joseph Y. Porter to Willard Knowlton, January 6, 1915, RG 894, Series 46, Box 28, Folder 6, State Archives of Florida, Tallahassee, FL (hereinafter SAF). I will discuss Porter in greater depth in Chapter 3.

2. Willard Knowlton to Joseph Y. Porter, January 12, 1915, RG 894, Series 46, Box 28, Folder 6, SAF. Unfortunately, the attached prints were not saved in the archives.

3. Joseph Y. Porter to Willard Knowlton, January 15, 1915, RG 894, Series 46, Box 28, Folder 6, SAF.

4. Julie K. Brown, *Health and Medicine on Display: International Expositions in the United States, 1876–1904* (Cambridge, MA: MIT Press, 2009), 65–76; Lynne Curry, *Modern Mothers in the Heartland: Gender, Health, and Progress in Illinois, 1900–1930* (Columbus: Ohio State University Press, 1999), chap. 4; Janet Golden, "The Iconography of Child Public Health: Between Medicine and Reform," in *Children's Health Issues in Historical Perspective*, ed. Cheryl Kranick Warsh and Veronic Strong-Boag (Waterloo, Ontario, Canada: Wilfrid Laurier University Press, 2005), 391–407.

5. "Great European Exhibit Expert Joins the Panama Pacific Exposition Forces," *Flaming Sword* XXVIII, (June 1914): 182.

6. Brown, *Health and Medicine on Display*, 25–29 and 60–63. On precedent, see Michael Sappol, *A Traffic of Dead Bodies: Anatomy and Embodied Social Identity in Nineteenth-Century America* (Princeton, NJ: Princeton University Press, 2002), chap. 9.

7. E. G. Routzahn to Ernst Meyer, September 19, 1914, Rockefeller Foundation Records (hereinafter RF), RG 5 International Health Board/Division Records (hereinafter IHB/D) 1.1, Box 9, Folder 146, Rockefeller Archive Center, Tarrytown, NY (hereinafter RAC). Routzahn's list in order was as follows: V. E. Baillard, 18 Frankfort, New York City; Mazie O. Barnes, 37 Emory Street, Jersey City, New Jersey; H. E. Boucher, 150 Lafayette Street, New York City; De Hart Mfg. Co. 418 West 27th Street, New York City; Einson, 813 Broadway; Educational Exhibit Company, Providence, Rhode Island; Le Lash Studios, Long Acre Building, 42nd St. and Broadway; Morgan Bros., Grand Central Palace, New York City; Royal Rook, 34 Pine Street, New York City; Edward Unitt, 142 West 46th Street, New York City; Herr Rauer, 9 Naunhoferstrasse, Marienhohe, Leipzig, Germany.

8. Ernst Meyer to E. G. Routzahn, October 24, 1914, RF RG 5 IHB/D 1.1, Box 9, Folder 146, RAC. Meyer added: Mr. Victor Mindeleff, 3033 P Street, N.W. Washington, D.C. and Howell's Microcosm, Washington, D.C.

9. The arguments made by the various contemporary body exhibits in defense of displaying life or lifelike elements that are simultaneously sanitized to avoid creating offense are reminiscent of those expressed by early twentieth-century health officials and reformers. However, I have yet to find debates about the ethics of putting bodies on display, a topic of contemporary concern, in this earlier period. I believe there are two reasons for this. First, the bodies on display in public health exhibits were not actual cadavers. (I will explain this in greater depth later in this chapter.)

Second, the practice of putting disabled bodies on display as a form of popular amusement was indicative of a widespread acceptance of this form of presentation. See, for instance, Charleen M. Moore and C. Mackenzie Brown, "Experiencing *Body Worlds*: Voyeurism, Education, or Enlightenment?" *Journal of Medical Humanities* 28, no. 4 (Winter 2007): 231–54, and Andrea Stulman Dennett, *Weird and Wonderful: The Dime Museum in America* (New York: New York University Press, 1997), especially chap. 4.

10. John Ettling, *The Germ of Laziness: Rockefeller Philanthropy and Public Health in the New South* (Cambridge, MA: Harvard University Press, 1981), chap. 8. On the development of the International Health Division, see John Farley, *To Cast Out Disease: A History of the International Health Division of the Rockefeller Foundation (1913–1951)* (Oxford: Oxford University Press, 2004).

11. Brown, *Health and Medicine on Display*, 63.

12. Erin McLeary and Elizabeth Toon, "Here Man Learns about Himself," *American Journal of Public Health* 102, no. 7 (July 2012): e28–e30.

13. Klaus Vogel, "The Transparent Man—Some Comments on the History of a Symbol," in *Manifesting Medicine: Bodies and Machines*, ed. Robert Bud, Bernard Finn, and Helmuth Trischler (Amsterdam: Harwood Academic, 1999), 37–38; Elena Canadelli, "'Scientific Peep Show': The Human Body in Contemporary Science Museums," *Nuncius* 26 (2011): 166.

14. McLeary and Toon, "Here Man Learns about Himself," e31–e34.

15. "Health Conservation at the Panama-Pacific Exposition," *New England Medical Gazette* XLX, no. 3 (March 1915): 164; "Great European Exhibit Expert Joins the Panama Pacific Exposition Forces," *Flaming Sword* XXVIIL (June 1914): 182 and 295. After much scouring, I have been unable to unearth any other records than what I have included related to Rauer that might shed light on his personal life before and after migrating to the United States.

16. Ernst Meyer to Philipp Rauer, October 4, 1915, RF RG5 IHB/D S1.1, Box 9, Folder 141, Rockefeller Archive Center, Sleepy Hollow, New York, RAC.

17. Ernst Meyer to Philipp Rauer, June 23, 1914, RF RG5 IHB/D S1.1, Box 8, Folder 137, RAC. Calculation of relative value done with measuringworth.com.

18. "Great European Exhibit Expert Joins the Panama Pacific Exposition Forces," *Flaming Sword* XXVIIL (June 1914): 295.

19. Ibid.

20. "Health Conservation at the Panama-Pacific Exposition," *New England Medical Gazette* XLX, no. 3 (March 1915): 164.

21. Memorandum on the Exhibit on Hookworm Disease Installed by the International Health Commission at the Panama-Pacific International Exposition at San Francisco, California, January 26, 1916, RF RG 5 IHB/D S Ss205 California, Box 6 Folder 41, RAC.

22. Ettling, *The Germ of Laziness*, chap. 5.

23. William A. Link, "Privies, Progressivism, and Public Schools: Health Reform and Education in the Rural South, 1909–1920," *Journal of Southern History* 54, no. 4 (November 1988): 640.

24. Ernst Meyer to C. W. Stiles, June 23, 1914, RF RG5 IHB/D S1.1, Box 8, Folder 137, RAC.

25. Ibid.

26. Ernst Meyer to C. W. Stiles, June 27, 1914, RF RG5 IHB/D S1.1, Box 8, Folder 137, RAC.

27. Agreement between the International Health Commission and Philipp Rauer, June 26, 1914, RF RG5 IHB/D S1.1, Box 8 Folder, Folder 137, RAC.

28. Memorandum on the Payment of $1,000 to Dr. Rauer in Connection with the Preparation of Wax Models, June 26, 1914, RF RG5 IHB/D S1.1, Box, 8, Folder 137, RAC.

29. C. W. Stiles to Ernst Meyer, July 7, 1914, RF RG5 HB/D S1.1, Box, 8, Folder 138, RAC.

30. Petit Cash Account International Health Commission for June and July 1914, RF RG5 IHB/D S1.1, Box 10, Folder 154, RAC.

31. Johns Hopkins Hospital Abstract of Record for Selma Ellis, May 2, 1915, RF RG5 IHB/D S1.1, Box 3, Folder 42–E1, RAC.

32. "Work of Hookworm Dispensaries," *Caucasian* (Cinto, NC), October 12, 1911.

33. "How to Improve Race in Morals," *Times Dispatch* (Richmond, VA), September 21, 1912.

34. "View Hookworm Victim," *Philadelphia Inquirer* (Philadelphia, PA), September 21, 1912.

35. "Free Treatment for Hookworm Disease," *Watauga Democrat* (Watauga, NC), October 24, 1912; "How Hookworm Disease Is Contracted," *Pickens Sentinel* (Pickens, SC), October 24, 1912.

36. Telegram from C. W. Stiles to Ernst Meyer, June 29, 1914, RF RG5 IHB/D S1.1, Box 8, Folder 137, RAC.

37. C. W. Stiles to Ernst Meyer, June 30, 1914, RF RG5 IHB/D S1.1, Box 8, Folder 137, RAC.

38. Philipp Rauer to Ernst Meyer, July 1, 1914, RF RG5 IHB/D S1.1, Box 8, Folder 138, RAC.

39. C. W. Stiles to Ernst Meyer, July 11, 1914, RF RG5 IHB/D S1.1, Box 10, Folder 154, RAC.

40. C. W. Stiles to Ernst Meyer, June 30, 1914, RF RG5 IHB/D S1.1, Box 8, Folder 137, RAC.

41. Petit Cash Account International Health Commission for June and July 1914, RF RG5 S1.1, Box 10, Folder 154, RAC.

42. Selma Ellis to C. W. Stiles, December 27, 1914, RF RG5 IHB/D S1.1, Box 3, Folder 42-E1, RAC.

43. Ernst Meyer to C. W. Stiles, January 6, 1915, RF RG5 IHB/D S1.1, Box 3, Folder 42-E1, RAC.

44. C. W. Stiles to Ernst Meyer, January 7, 1915, RF RG5 IHB/D S1.1, Box 3, Folder 42-E1, RAC.

45. C. W. Stiles to Pelton Ellis, May 1, 1915, RF RG5 IHB/D S1.1, Box 3, Folder 42-E1, RAC.

46. Selma Ellis to Wickliffe Rose, June 1, 1915, RF RG5 IHB/D S1.1, Box 3, Folder 42-E1, RAC.

47. C. W. Stiles to Wickliffe Rose, June 4, 1915, RF RG 5 IHB/D S1.1, Box 3, Folder 42-E1, RAC.

48. For more on various constructions of underserving and deserving poor in the early twentieth century, see Linda Gordon, *Pitied but Not Entitled: Single Mothers and the History of Welfare* (New York: Free Press, 1994).

49. In 1917, Selma Ellis was working as a farmer, but his leg was still an issue. He applied for an exemption from military service during World War I because of an "ulcer on leg 14 years." World War I Draft Registration Cards, 1917–1918, ancestry.com.

50. Philipp Rauer to Ernst Meyer, July 6, 1914, RF RG5 IHB/D S1.1, Box 8, Folder 138, RAC.

51. Alvin E. Pope to Philipp Rauer, June 27, 1914 and E. B. Barnet to Philipp Rauer, June 27, 1914, RF RG5 IHB/D S1.1, Box 8, Folder 138, RAC.

52. Alvin E. Pope to Ernst Meyer, July 9, 1914, RF RG5 IHB/D S1.1, Box 8, Folder 138, RAC.

53. Ernst Meyer to C. W. Stiles, June 29, 1914, RF RG5 IHB/D S1.1, Box 8, Folder 137, RAC.

54. Sterling Bunnell was a mechanical engineer. I have not been able to unearth any archival records that indicate how they became acquainted. On Bunnell, see http://hdl.handle.net/10079/fa/mssa.ms.1149.

55. J. B. Gantz to Ernst Meyer, September 19, 1914, and September 20, 1914, RF RG5 IHB/D 1.1, Box 9, Folder 139; Ernst Meyer to J. B. Gantz, September 22, 1914, RF RG5 IHB/D 1.1, Box 9, Folder 139, RAC.

56. Sterling H. Bunnell to Wickliffe Rose, September 24, 1914, RF RG5 IHB/D 1.1, Box 9, Folder 139.

57. J. B. Gantz to Ernst Meyer, September 19, 1914, RF RG5 IHB/D 1.1, Box 9, Folder 139. Philipp Rauer to Ernst Meyer, August 31, 1914, RF RG5 IHB/D 1.1, Box 9, Folder 139, translation by Christian Juergens. Rauer arrived in the United States on June 13, 1914, fifteen days before Archduke Franz Ferdinand was assassinated. After the war broke out, Rauer declared his intention to become a U.S. citizen. See Philipp Robert Jusef Rauer, Petition for Naturalization, October 13, 1914, ancestry.com.

58. John A. Ferrell to H. W. Rose, June 18, 1940, RF RG2-1940, Series 200, Box 191, Folder 1364, RAC.

59. Ernst Meyer to Philipp Rauer, January 8, 1915, RF RG5 IHB/D S1.1, Box 9, Folder 141, RAC.

60. Ernst Meyer to Philipp Rauer, April 21, 1915, RF RG5 IHB/D S1.1, Box 9, Folder 141, RAC.

61. Jessica B. Peixotto, "San Francisco: What the Panama-Pacific Exposition Promises to a Social Worker," *Survey* 34, no. 14 (July 3, 1915): 310–11.

62. Ernst Meyer to Philipp Rauer, May 4, 1917, RF RG5 IHB/D S1.1, Box 25 Folder 425, RAC.

63. Ernst Meyer to Whom It May Concern, June 1, 1915, RF RG5 IHB/D S1.1, Box 9, Folder 141, RAC.

64. Memorandum for Dr. W. H. Tolman of the American Museum of Safety, New York City, for Use in the Preparation of a Description of Models on Hookworm Disease Prepared by Dr. Philipp Rauer and for Use in the Bulletin "Safety" of the Museum, December 14, 1914, RF RG5 IHB/D S1.1, Box 9, Folder 140, RAC.

65. Ibid.

66. Ibid.

67. Ibid.

68. Ernst Meyer to Alvin Pope, May 20, 1915, RF RG5 IHB/D S1.1, Box 19, Folder 294, RAC.

69. Memorandum for Dr. W. H. Tolman of the American Museum of Safety, New York City, for Use in the Preparation of a Description of Models on Hookworm Disease Prepared by Dr. Philipp Rauer and for Use in the Bulletin "Safety" of the Museum, December 14, 1914, RF RG5 IHB/D S1.1, Box 9, Folder 140, RAC.

70. Ibid.

71. News of Rauer's arrival in the United States made the papers. See "Biggest Liner Has No Trouble Docking," *New York Sun*, June 13, 1914.

72. Letter from Philipp Rauer to Joseph Y. Porter, January 5, 1915, RG 894, Series 46, Box 28, Folder 6, SAF.

73. Ibid.

74. Ibid.

75. For more on the museum's history, see Ross Wilson, "The Museum of Safety: Responsibility, Awareness and Modernity in New York, 1909–1923," *Journal of American Studies* 51, no. 3 (2017): 915–38.

76. "Shoes and Feet," *Safety* 3, no. 8 (1915): 204.

77. Ibid., 205.

78. Ibid.

79. Ibid.

80. Ibid.

81. "Incorporations, Secretary of State," *Weekly Reports and Index: Decisions, Opinions and Rulings, New York State Departments Commissions and Courts*, 1: 39.

82. "Capital Increases," *New York Times*, December 18, 1917.

83. Official Gazette, United States Patent Office, CCLXXV (June 1920): 112.

84. Advertisement, *New York Central Lines Industrial Directory and Shipper's Guide* (1920–1921): 383.

85. Judgments (the first name is of the debtor) Business Records, *New York Times*, May 7, 1935.

86. "Building in Queens Bought from Bank," *New York Times*, September 25, 1941.

87. "Offer of 'Cortisone' in Bulk Traps Three Here on Charges of Fraud," *New York Times*, August 11, 1951; "Arrests Trio in Illegal Sale of Scare Drug," *Brooklyn New York Daily Eagle*, August 11, 1951.

88. "Offer of 'Cortisone' in Bulk Traps Three Here on Charges of Fraud," *New York Times*, August 11, 1951.

89. Letters from Mica Heidemann to Dr. Brown Goode, May 6, 1885, RG 189, Box 53, Folder 7, Smithsonian Institution Archives, Washington D.C., "Reports, News Items, Notes," *Kindergarten Museum* XIII, no. 1 (September, 1900): 51; *Report on the Progress and Condition of the U.S. National Museum for the Year Ending June 30, 1907* (Washington, D.C.: Government Printing Office, 1907), 86. Everything I have been unable to unearth about Mica Heidemann's personal and professional life is contained within this chapter.

90. "Otto Heidemann," *Entomological News* 28, no. 1 (1917): 1–2.

91. "Agricultural Department," *Evening Times*, Washington, D.C., October 4, 1902; Harry B. Weiss and Grace M. Ziegler, "Notes on Some Wood Engravers of North American Insects," *Journal of the New York Entomological Society* 36, no. 4 (December 1928): 427. Otto Heidemann died in Washington, D.C. on November 17, 1916.

92. Ibid.

93. Ibid.

94. Ibid.

95. A. G. Wheeler Jr., Thomas J. Henry, and Thomas L. Mason Jr., "An Annotated List of the Miridae of West Virginia (Hemiptera-Heteroptera)," *Transactions of the American Entomological Society* 109, no. 1 (1983): 129.

96. Ibid.

97. Virgil E. McMahan, "Mica Zester Heidemann," in *The Artists of Washington, D.C.* (Washington, DC: Government Printing Office, 1995).

98. The Office of the Surgeon General to Joseph Y. Porter, January 17, 1916, RG 894, Series 46, Box 29, Folder 8, SAF.

99. "Making Gigantic Bugs," *Sun*, October 7, 1906.

100. Ibid.

101. "Financial Statement for Fiscal Year, August 1, 1904 to August 1, 1905," *Tenth Annual Report of the State Entomologist of Minnesota to the Governor for the Year 1905*: xv. For the relative value, see www.measuringworth.com.

102. University of the State of New York, *Education Department Bulletin*, Report No. 455 (September 15, 1909): 10.

103. The Office of the Surgeon General to Joseph Y. Porter, January 17, 1916, RG 894, Series 46, Box 29, Folder 8, SAF.

104. Joseph Y. Porter to Mrs. Otto Heidemann, January 22, 1916, RG 894, Series 46, Box 29, Folder 8, SAF; Mrs. Otto Heidemann to Joseph Y. Porter with pamphlet included, January 25, 1916, RG 894, Series 46, Box 29, Folder 8, SAF.

105. Obituary, "Otto Heidemann," *Washington Post*, November 21, 1916.

106. Heidemann remained in Schenectady until her death in the early 1930s. Search "Mica Heidemann" ancestry.com (Information in City Directories and 1930 census). The last record is a listing in the city's directory for 1931.

107. Swarts Jr. did not leave much by way of a personal archival trail. According to the 1910, 1920, and 1930 censuses, he continued to live with his parents into adulthood (his father had died by the 1930 census, but his mother was still alive). Each census listed his occupation as a civil engineer. Swarts was born in 1885. He graduated from Harvard in 1907. See "Gardner T. Swarts Jr.," obituary in the *New York Times* on October 22, 1934. He wrote about himself in a report to Harvard for its third report. *Harvard College (1780–) Class of 1907, Third Report* (1910): 293, https://books.google.com/books?id=nsgnAAAAYAAJ&dq=gardner%20swarts%20harvard%20third%20report&pg=PA293#v=onepage&q=gardner%20swarts%20harvard%20third%20report&f=false.

108. Gardner T. Swarts Jr. to Joseph Y. Porter, October 24, 1914, RG 894, Series 46, Box 28, Folder 3, SAF.

109. *Harvard College (1780–) Class of 1907, Third Report* (1910): 293–94, https://books.google.com/books?id=nsgnAAAAYAAJ&dq=gardner%20swarts%20harvard%20third%20report&pg=PA293#v=onepage&q=gardner%20swarts%20harvard%20third%20report&f=false. *Harvard College (1780–) Class of 1907, Fourth Report* (1917): 430, https://books.google.com/books?id=CcknAAAAYAAJ&dq=robert%20gowen%20harvard%20fourth%20report&pg=PA429#v=onepage&q=robert%20gowen%20harvard%20fourth%20report&f=false.

110. After much scouring, I have been unable to locate any archival company records for the Educational Exhibition Company.

111. *Educational Exhibitions, Catalogue C* (Educational Exhibition Co., 1914).

112. *Public Health Exhibitions: A Catalogue of Necessaries for Their Outfitting and Maintenance, Catalogue B* (Educational Exhibition Co., August 1910), 2.

113. Ibid., 20.

114. *Educational Exhibitions, Catalogue C* (Educational Exhibition Co., 1914), 12.

115. Ibid.,14.

116. *Public Health Exhibitions: A Catalogue of Necessaries for Their Outfitting and Maintenance, Catalogue B* (Educational Exhibition Co., August 1910), 8.

117. *Educational Exhibitions, Catalogue C* (Educational Exhibition Co., 1914), 57.

118. *Public Health Exhibitions: A Catalogue of Necessaries for Their Outfitting and Maintenance, Catalogue B* (Educational Exhibition Co., August 1910), 13.

119. Ibid., 28.

120. Ibid., 26.

121. *Public Health Exhibitions: A Catalogue of Necessaries for Their Outfitting and Maintenance, Catalogue B* (Educational Exhibition Co., August 1910), 13.

122. Ibid.

123. Ibid., 14.

124. *Educational Exhibitions, Catalogue C* (Educational Exhibition Co., 1914), 65.

125. State Board of Health of Florida, *Twenty-Seventh Annual Report of the State Board of Health of Florida* (1915): 24.

126. Joseph Y. Porter to J. E. Taylor, November 11, 1914, RG 894, Series 46, Box 28, Folder 4, SAF.

127. Gardner T. Swarts Jr. to Joseph Y. Porter, October 7, 1914, RG 894, Series 46, Box 28, Folder 3, SAF.

128. Gardner T. Swarts Jr. to Joseph Y. Porter, December 2, 1914, RG 894, Series 46, Box 28, Folder 5, SAF.

129. "Interview on Friday, Dec. 10, 1914," RG 894, Series 46, Box 28, Folder 5, SAF.

130. Joseph Y. Porter to Gardner T. Swarts Jr., October 25, 1914, RG 894, Series 46, Box 28, Folder 3, SAF; Joseph Y. Porter to Gardner T. Swarts Jr., November 6, 1914, RG 894, Series 46, Box 28, Folder 4, SAF.

131. Gardner T. Swarts Jr. to Joseph Y. Porter, October 19, 1914, RG 894, Series 46, Box 28, Folder 3, SAF.

132. Swarts's fortunes were cut short when, in 1934 at the age of fifty, he died. It does not appear that his company continued without him. Obituary, "Gardner T. Swarts Jr.," *New York Times*, October 22, 1934.

133. "Evart G. Routzahn," Russell Sage Foundation Records (hereinafter RSF), Series 2, Box 2, Folder 18, RAC; Obituary: "Evart Routzahn," *New York Times*, April 25, 1939, RSF, Series 2, Box 2, Folder 18, RAC. I have referenced everything about Routzahn's personal and professional life that I have been able to find in this chapter.

134. "Announcement of the Retirement of Evart G. Routzahn," June 22, 1934, RSF, Series 3, Box 33, Folder 266, RAC.

135. Ibid.

136. At Routzahn's death in 1939, the *American Journal of Public Health* described him as an "apostle of health." "Evart Grant Routzahn," *American Journal of Public Health* 29, no. 6 (June 1939): 655; RSF, Series 2, Box 2, Folder 18, RAC. His peers described him as "a pioneer" and as "a prodder, a stimulator, a teacher who taught by clinic and example, not by dogma." Obituary, "Evart Grant Routzahn," *New York School News*, May 1939, RSF, Series 2, Box 2, Folder 18, RAC; "Evart Grant Routzahn," *Channels*, May 1939 RSF, Series 2, Box 2, Folder 18, RAC. Harrison asserted that Routzahn "knew the importance of making material interesting, simple, graphic, and colorful, while at the same time sticking to ascertained facts." Florence M. Seder, who wrote the obituary for the news bulletin of the Social Work Publicity Council, said "[Routzahn] loved the fresh and vivid approach, the crystal-clear wording, the color in which an old truth might be newly dressed." "Evart Grant Routzahn," *Channels*, May 1939 RSF, Series 2, Box 2, Folder 18, RAC. According to Harrison, Routzahn understood that "showmanship" was necessary to "improv[e] people's health and well being." "Evart G. Routzahn," RSF, Series 2, Box 2, Folder 18, RAC.

137. "Evart Grant Routzahn Passes on in New York; Began Work in Tuberculosis Thirty-Five Years Ago," *Bulletin of the National Tuberculosis Association*, June 1939, RSF, Series 3, Box 33, Folder 266, RAC.

138. Ibid.

139. "Obituary: Evart Routzahn, Social Worker, 70," *New York Times*, April 25, 1939; RSF, Series 2, Box 2, Folder 18, RAC.

140. "Evart Grant Routzahn," *Channels*, May 1939 RSF, Series 2, Box 2, Folder 18, RAC.

141. "Evart Grant Routzahn Passes on in New York; Began Work in Tuberculosis Thirty-Five Years Ago," *Bulletin of the National Tuberculosis Association*, June 1939, RSF, Series 3, Box 33, Folder 266, RAC.

142. E. G. Routzahn, "The Value of the Tuberculosis Exhibition," *Survey* 23 (November 20, 1909): 253.

143. Ibid.

144. Ibid.

145. Ibid.

146. Ibid.

147. Ibid.

148. "A National Clearing-House for Social Surveys and Exhibits," *Survey* 29 (October 5, 1912): 1.

149. E. G. Routzahn to National Associations and Others, November 30, 1912, RF RG 5 IHB/D 1.1 Box 9, Folder 146, RAC.

150. Ibid.

151. "Cycle of Child Life Shown by Welfare League at the Peoria Exhibition," *Survey* 29 (January 3, 1913): 372.

152. "Biographical Notes about Mrs. Mary Swain Routzahn," October 26, 1944; RSF, Series 2, Box 2, Folder 18, RAC.

153. "Brief Course in Publicity," *Survey* 65 (March 15, 1931).

154. Leon Whipple, "The Routzahns Tell Everything," *Survey* 60 (June 15, 1928): 353.

155. E. G. Routzahn, "Second International Exposition of Safety and Sanitation," December 17, 1914, RF RG 5 IHB/D 1.1, Box 9, Folder 146, RAC.

156. E. G. Routzahn to J. A. Farrell, May 11, 1915, RF RG 5 IHB/D 1.1, Box 9, Folder 146, RAC.

157. Evart G. Routzahn and Mary Swain Routzahn, "Why Have an Exhibit," *Survey* 40 (July 27, 1918): 474.

158. Ibid.

159. Ibid.

160. Ibid., 473.

161. Department of Surveys and Exhibitions, Russell Sage Foundation, "Plan for the Study of Social Welfare Publicity," November 3, 1919, RSF, Series 3, Box 33, Folder 264, RAC.

162. Ibid.

163. Ibid.

164. Evart G. Routzahn and Mary Swain Routzahn, *The A B C of Exhibit Planning* (New York: Russell Sage Foundation, 1918), 4.

165. Leon Whipple, "The Routzahns Tell Everything," *Survey* 60 (June 15, 1928): 353.

166. Ibid.

167. Ibid.

168. Routzahn, *The A B C of Exhibit Planning*, 1.

169. Ibid., 22.

170. Ibid.

171. Ibid., 31.

172. Ibid., 43.

173. Ibid., 15.

174. Ibid., 57.

175. Ibid., 71.

176. Ibid.

177. On the use of photography to make an argument in the Progressive Era, see Kate Sampsell Willmann, "Lewis Hine, Ellis Island, and Pragmatism: Photographs as Lived Experience," *Journal of the Gilded Age and Progressive Era* 7, no. 2 (April 2008): 221–52.

178. Memo dated May 1, 1934, RSF, Series 3, Box 33, Folder 266, RAC.

3. Health Trains

1. Public Health Published by the Michigan State Board of Health (1913): 28, Box 6, Lee Barnett Collection, Clarke Historical Library, Central Michigan University.

2. Ibid.

3. John Duffy, *The Sanitarians: A History of American Public Health* (Urbana: University of Illinois Press, 1990), chaps. 13–15.

4. Jennifer Koslow, *Cultivating Health: Los Angeles Women and Public Health Reform* (New Brunswick, NJ: Rutgers University Press, 2009), chap. 3.

5. A variety of states used health trains between 1911 and 1931. See "Michigan, Health Train Starts," *JAMA* 57, no. 6 (1911): 488; "Iowa, Health Train for Iowa," *JAMA* 57, no. 7 (1911): 569; "Colorado, Health Train for Colorado," *JAMA* 57, no. 8 (1911): 662; "Kentucky, State Health Car," *JAMA* 57, no. 14 (1911): 1142; "Virginia, Health Train," *JAMA* 58, no. 9 (1911): 644; "Maryland, Tuberculosis Exhibit," *JAMA* 58, no. 12 (1912): 867; "Kansas, Health Car," *JAMA* 73, no. 18 (1919): 1369; "Arkansas, Health Train Starts," *JAMA* 75, no. 1 (1920): 40; "Texas, Educational Campaign against Malaria," *JAMA* 75, no. 14 (1920): 946; "Georgia, Train Called 'The Hygienian,'" *JAMA* 96, no. 18 (1931): 1514. Even Canada tried the experiment; see "Quebec," *Canadian Medical Association Journal* 11, no. 11 (November 1921): 872, http://www.ncbi.nlm.nih.gov/pmc/articles/PMC1524402/pdf/canmedaj00410-0090.pdf.

6. Julie K. Brown, "'. . . Touching the Life of the City of New York': The American Museum of Natural History and Exhibiting Modern Health in the early Progressive Era," paper, Annual Conference American Association for the History of Medicine, Rochester, New York, 2010; "Thousands at the Tuberculosis Exhibit," *Charities and The Commons* XV, no. 10 (1905): 345; "Tuberculosis Exhibition in Chicago," *Charities and The Commons* XVI, no. 2 (April 14, 1906): 91.

7. May 21, 1907, Minutes of the State Board of Health, California, Department of Public Health Records R384.001 (F3676:1–27a, F3676:30–89)/Minutes (1903–1973), California State Archives, Sacramento (hereinafter CSA).

8. Ibid.

9. August 27, 1908, and December 4, 1908, Minutes of the State Board of Health, California, Department of Public Health Records R384.001 (F3676:1–27a, F3676:30–89)/Minutes (1903–1973), CSA; regarding the American Tuberculosis Exhibition's inspiration for the California Sanitation Car, see also California State Board of Health, *The Sanitation Car* (Sacramento: California State Board of Health, May 1911), 2, California History Room, California State Library, Sacramento (hereinafter CSL); Thomas McNeese Keller, "Public Health on the Railroad: William Freeman Snow and the California Sanitation Exhibit," *American Journal of Public Health* 87, no. 11 (November 1997): 1859–61.

10. LeRoy Barnett, "Putting Michigan Farmers on the Right Track," *Michigan History Magazine*, January/February 2000, 50–51.

11. A search of "corn gospel train" in two newspaper databases, America's Historical Newspapers and Chronicling America, indicates that newspapers around the nation covered this story. Californians could read about it in the May 17, 1905, issue of the *San Francisco Call*.

12. According to the U.S. Census, California's total population in 1910 was 2,377,549 (rural 907,810 [33.2 percent]; urban 1,469,739 [61.8 percent]). U.S. Bureau of the Census, *Thirteenth Census of the United States: 1910 Volume 4; Population 1910* (Washington, D.C.: Government Printing Office), 140, http://www.census.gov/prod/www /decennial.html. The U.S. Census classified the majority of residents in both urban and rural areas in 1910 as white (almost 96 percent for urban areas and almost 94 percent for rural areas). African Americans numbered 1 percent of urban dwellers and less than 1 percent of rural dwellers. "Indian, Chinese, and Japanese" constituted 3 percent of urban dwellers and almost 6 percent of rural dwellers. Foreign-born whites constituted 41 percent of the state's urban population and 35 percent of its rural population. Foreign-born differed upon location. In 1920, for instance, the U.S. Census calculated that in Los Angeles, the largest group of foreign-born whites was from Mexico (19.3 percent). In San Francisco, the largest group was from Ireland (18 percent). U.S. Bureau of the Census, "California: Table 1. Color or Race, Nativity, Percentage, and Sex for the State and Urban and Rural Population: 1920, 1910, and 1900," in *Fourteenth Census of the United States Taken in the Year 1920, Volume 3: Population 1920: Composition and Characteristics of the Population by States* (Washington, D.C.: Government Printing Office), 106, and U.S. Bureau of the Census, "California: Table 6. Country of Birth of the Foreign-Born White, for the State and Principal Cities: 1920," in *Fourteenth Census of the United States Taken in the Year 1920, Volume 3: Population 1920: Composition and Characteristics of the Population by States* (Washington, D.C.: Government Printing Office), 109.

13. Koslow, *Cultivating Health*, chap. 3.

14. "Health Car to Cover State," *Los Angeles Times*, December 15, 1908.

15. Quoted in W. F. Snow, "The California Sanitation Exhibit" (1909): 111 in H. O. Jenkins, "A Traveling Sanitation Exhibit Directed by the State Board of Health of California in 1909," (1910), CSL.

16. See Duffy, *The Sanitarians*, 223; John Ettling, *The Germ of Laziness: Rockefeller Philanthropy and Public Health in the New South* (Cambridge, MA: Harvard University Press, 1981); Judith Sealander, *Private Wealth and Public Life, Foundation Philanthropy and the Reshaping of American Social Policy from the Progressive Era to the New Deal* (Baltimore: Johns Hopkins University Press, 1997), 59–67; William A. Link, "Privies, Progressivism, and Public Schools: Health Reform and Education in the Rural South, 1909–1920," *Journal of Southern History* 54, no. 4 (November 1988): 623–42. On the limited influence of philanthropy on southern public health among mill towns, see Edward H. Beardsley, *A History of Neglect: Health Care for Blacks and Mill Workers in the Twentieth-Century South* (Knoxville: University of Tennessee Press, 1987), 51–54. On philanthropic involvement in professionalizing public health in the twentieth century, see Fee, *Disease & Discovery*, especially chap. 2.

17. H. O. Jenkins, "A Traveling Sanitation Exhibit Directed by the State Board of Health of California in 1909" (1910), 4, CSL.

18. Guenter B. Risse, *Plague, Fear, and Politics, in San Francisco's Chinatown* (Baltimore: Johns Hopkins University Press, 2012), 127–30.

19. Jenkins, "A Traveling Sanitation Exhibit," 4.

20. Andrew Carnegie, "Wealth," *North American Review* 148, no. 391 (June 1889): 661–62.

21. June 25, 1909, Minutes of the State Board of Health, California, Department of Public Health Records R384.001 (F3676:1–27a, F3676:30–89)/Minutes (1903–1973), CSA.

22. "'Health Car' to Visit San Jose," *Evening News* (San Jose, CA), March 31, 1909; "Health Car to Be Shown Here," *Evening News* (San Jose, CA), April 16, 1909. The students were only ever identified as "several students of Stanford University" without specifics to a degree program. See also the section "The Plan" from the pamphlet entitled "The California Sanitation Exhibit" (1909), included in H. Jenkins, "A Traveling Sanitation Exhibit," CSL.

23. On tuberculosis in California, see Emily Abel, *Politics of Exclusion: A History of Public Health and Migration to Los Angeles* (New Brunswick, NJ: Rutgers University Press, 2007); Emily Abel, *Suffering in the Land of Sunshine: A Los Angeles Illness Narrative* (New Brunswick, NJ: Rutgers University Press, 2006); Natalia Molina, *Fit to Be Citizens? Public Health and Race in Los Angeles* (Berkeley: University of California Press, 2006).

24. See section "The Plan" from the pamphlet entitled "The California Sanitation Exhibit" (1909), included in H. Jenkins, "A Traveling Sanitation Exhibit," CSL.

25. Abel, *Tuberculosis and Politics of Exclusion*, 30–31 and chap. 6.

26. California State Board of Health, *The Sanitation Car* (no. 13), 6, CSL.

27. California State Board of Health, *The Sanitation Car* (no. 13), 6, CSL; August 27, 1908, Minutes of the State Board of Health, California, Department of Public Health Records R384.001 (F3676:1–27a, F3676:30–89)/Minutes (1903–1973), CSA.

28. The U.S. Bureau of the Census, "California. Chapter 2 Composition and Characteristics of the Population," in *Thirteenth Census of the United States Taken in the Year 1910, Volume 2: Population 1910: Reports by States for Counties, Cities, and Other Civil Divisions* (Washington, D.C.: Government Printing Office), 156.

29. Ibid. The percentages of illiteracy for various subsets were foreign-born whites (10 percent), African Americans (7.1 percent), Indians (49 percent), Chinese (15.5 percent), and Japanese (8.6 percent). Rural areas also had a higher percentage of illiteracy than urban areas (5.9 percent versus 2.4 percent).

30. The most extensive set of images was included in a report by H. O. Jenkins. Jenkins was a graduate of Stanford and an "assistant in the biological department of the Massachusetts Institute of Technology." Regarding Jenkins's biographical information, see *Sixth Annual Report of the President of the University*, for year ending July 31, 1909, Stanford University, 50, accessed via Google books: https://books.google.com/books ?id=cm8-AAAAYAAJ&lpg=RA5-PA50&ots=NH5xFoitfC&dq=H.O.%20Jenkins%20 Massachusetts%20Institute%20of%20Technology&pg=RA4-PA54#v=onepage&q =Jenkins%20&f=false. Jenkins later became Palo Alto's health officer.

31. Jenkins, "A Traveling Sanitation Exhibit" (no. 20), Fig. 5, CSL.

32. Ibid.

33. "Health Car to Cover State," *Los Angeles Times*, December 15, 1908. On the use of female technicians at various world's fairs to demonstrate to viewers the process of examining food for microscopic disease, see Brown, *Health and Medicine on Display*, 110 and 115.

34. "Campaign for Sanitation Waged in State Board of Health Car," *San Francisco Call*, April 4, 1909.

35. Jenkins, "A Traveling Sanitation Exhibit" (no. 20), 10, CSL. Slide lectures were a popular way to convey educational health messages. See Golden, "The Iconography of Child Public Health," 391–407.

36. Newspaper accounts of the California train do not provide more than a description of the exhibit and the numbers who visited.

37. "Health Exhibit Car Visited by Hundreds," *Los Angeles Herald*, May 15, 1909.

38. "Health Car's Travels," *Los Angeles Times*, May 29, 1909.

39. "Campaign for Sanitation Waged in State Board of Health Car," *San Francisco Call*, April 4, 1909.

40. Jenkins, "A Traveling Sanitation Exhibit" (no. 20), 6, CSL. Unfortunately, newspapers and state officials did not record any qualitative descriptions of the reception of the exhibit by either rural or urban residents.

41. Ibid., 9.

42. Jenkins, "A Traveling Sanitation Exhibit" (no. 20), 9, CSL.

43. January 8, 1910, Minutes of the State Board of Health, California, Department of Public Health Records R384.001 (F3676:1–27a, F3676:30–89)/Minutes (1903–1973), CSA.

44. February 5, 1910, Minutes of the State Board of Health, California, Department of Public Health Records R384.001 (F3676:1–27a, F3676:30–89)/Minutes (1903–1973), CSA.

45. Gillett was not an enemy to the expansion of public health legislation. His inaugural address in 1907 supported the federal Pure Food Act. See http://governors.library.ca .gov/addresses/22-Gillett.html. I have been unable to find any specific archival evidence of Gillett's perspective about the train.

46. July 16, 1909, Minutes of the State Board of Health, California, Department of Public Health Records R384.001 (F3676:1–27a, F3676:30–89)/Minutes (1903–1973), CSA.

47. *The Twenty-First Biennial Report of the State Board of Health of California for the Fiscal Years from July 1, 1908 to June 30, 1910*, 245. Accessed via Google Books.

48. California State Board of Health, *The Sanitation Car* (no. 13), 8, CSL.

49. John Duffy offers a brief discussion of Louisiana's health train in Duffy, *The Sanitarians*, 226–27. As does Ettling, *Rockefeller Philanthropy*, 155, and Thomas Waisely; see Thomas Waisley, "Public Health Programs in Early Twentieth-Century Louisiana," *Louisiana History: The Journal of the Louisiana Historical Association* 41, no. 1 (Winter 2000): 58–60. Oscar Dowling was born in Montgomery, Alabama, on October 29, 1866. He received his medical degree from Vanderbilt University and obtained postgraduate training in New York, Chicago, London, Berlin, Paris, and Mexico. He returned to the South to start a practice with J. I. Darby in Columbus, Georgia. He later moved to Shreveport, Louisiana, setting up a specialty practice in eye, ear, nose, and throat cases. He became a member of the state's board of health in 1906 and became the institution's president in 1910. "Henry County News," *Columbus (Georgia) Enquirer-Sun*, February 15, 1889; "News and Gossip of Phoenix and Girard," *Columbus (Georgia) Enquirer-Sun*, September 9, 1902; Mike Miller, "Biography of Oscar Dowling, M.D., Montgomery, Alabama," http://files.usgwarchives.org/al/montgomery /bios/odowling.txt.

50. Oscar Dowling, "Health Conditions in Louisiana" (Louisiana State Board of Health, n.d.): front inset map; "Report of the President," in *Biennial Report of the Louisiana*

State Board of Health to the General Assembly of the State of Louisiana (1912–1913): front inset map. He brought the idea of a health train up upon his election to be president of the state board of health. See Minutes Books of the State Board of Health, September 20, 1910, page 333, P1978–136 5922A, Louisiana State Archives, Baton Rouge, LA (hereinafter LSA).

51. Charles V. Chapin, *A Report on State Public Health Work* (Chicago: American Medical Association, 1916), 163–64. On the inception of other trains, see note 5.

52. See speech by Henry Grady to northern investors from 1886, *Life and Labors of Henry W. Grady, His Speeches, Writings, Etc.* (Atlanta, GA: H. C. Hudgins & Co., 1890), 113, and Booker T. Washington's speech at the Atlanta Exposition in 1895. Booker T. Washington, *Up from Slavery* (New York: Doubleday, Page & Co., 1907), 219–20 and 222.

53. Frederick D. Mott and Milton I. Roemer, *Rural Health and Medical Care* (New York: McGraw-Hill, 1948), 7.

54. According to the U.S. Census, Louisiana's total population in 1910 was 1,656,388 (rural 1,159,872 [70 percent]; urban 496,516 [30 percent]). U.S. Bureau of the Census, *Thirteenth Census of the United States: 1910 Volume 4; Population 1910* (Washington, D.C.: Government Printing Office), http://www.census.gov/prod/www/decennial.html. The U.S. Census enumerated 56.8 percent of the state's population as white in 1910. Of that number, only 10 percent were foreign born. African Americans constituted 43.1 percent of the state's population in 1910. U.S. Bureau of the Census, "Louisiana. Chapter 2 Composition and Characteristics of the Population," in *Thirteenth Census of the United States Taken in the Year 1910, Volume 2: Population 1910: Reports by States for Counties, Cities, and Other Civil Divisions* (Washington, D.C.: Government Printing Office), 771.

55. Ibid., 333 and 339.

56. John Duffy argued that there were "few advances" in southern public health until the end of the nineteenth century. Duffy, *The Sanitarians*, 144. Alan Brinkley characterized Louisiana's public health facilities as "abysmal" before Huey Long taking office in 1928. Alan Brinkley, *Voices of Protest: Huey Long, Father Coughlin, and the Great Depression* (New York: Vintage, 1983), 30.

57. Margaret Humphreys, *Yellow Fever and the South* (New Brunswick, NJ: Rutgers University Press, 1992), 11 and 173.

58. Stuart Gallishoff, "Germs Know No Color Line: Black Health and Public Policy in Atlanta, 1900–1918," *Journal of the History of Medicine and Allied Sciences* 40, no. 1 (1985): 22–41, especially 33–39.

59. Ettling, *The Germ of Laziness*, 220.

60. Link, "Privies, Progressivism, and Public Schools," 623–42.

61. William A. Link, "'The Harvest Is Ripe, but the Laborers Are Few': The Hookworm Crusade in North Carolina, 1909–1915," *North Carolina Historical Review* 67, no. 1 (January 1990): 1–27, quotation on 15.

62. On the ubiquity of the circus, see Gregory J. Renoff, *The Big Tent: The Traveling Circus in Georgia, 1820–1930* (Athens: University of Georgia Press, 2008); Mark West, "A Spectrum of Spectators: Circus Audiences in Nineteenth-Century American," *Journal of Social History* 15, no. 2 (Winter 1981): 265–70.

63. Florida established a hookworm eradication program before the Rockefeller's venture. Hence, it did not participate in the Sanitary Commission program. Ettling, *The Germ of Laziness*, 123–24.

64. Ibid., 243.

65. "Report of the President," in *Biennial Report of the Louisiana State Board of Health to the General Assembly of the State of Louisiana* (1910–1911): 245–46, LSA.

66. Ibid., 244.

67. Ibid., 245.

68. Ibid., 27.

69. Ibid.

70. Ibid.

71. *Biennial Report of the Louisiana State Board of Health to the General Assembly of the State of Louisiana* (1910–1911): 30, LSA.

72. "A Health Exhibit on Wheels," *JAMA* 55, no. 18 (1910): 1560.

73. *Biennial Report of the Louisiana State Board of Health to the General Assembly of the State of Louisiana* (1910–1911): 27, LSA.

74. Ibid., 28.

75. "Criticism of the Health Train," *Times-Democratic*, March 9, 1911, Official Scrapbook #23, P1994-10, LSA.

76. "Report of the President," in *Louisiana Board of Health Report* (1912–1913): 123, P 1990-90/19115, LSA.

77. Ibid.

78. Ibid., 29. Unfortunately, unlike California, archival evidence of the objects in the Louisiana train is overwhelmingly textual. The few photographs that exist within copies of the state board of health's biennial reports and newspaper clippings are too grainy to make out details with any specificity.

79. Ibid., 28–29.

80. Ibid., 25; "Health on Wheels," *Southern Medical Journal* 43 (1911): 311–13.

81. "Health Train Arrives; Visited by Hundreds," *Macon Daily Telegraph*, December 6, 1914. The same exhibit showed up in Illinois; see Curry, *Modern Mothers*, 98.

82. "Health Train Arrives; Visited by Hundreds," *Macon Daily Telegraph*, December 6, 1914.

83. "Louisiana's Health Train," *Journal of the Outdoor Life: The Anti-Tuberculosis Magazine* 8, no. 8 (1911): 216. The Man Who Learned was about pure milk.

84. "Dowling's Health Train Will Be in City Today," *Montgomery Advertiser*, September 30, 1912.

85. "Report of the President," *Louisiana Board of Health Report* (1918–1919): 21, P 1990-90, LSA.

86. "Local Doctors Endorse Health Exhibit Train," *Macon Daily Telegraph*, December 3, 1914.

87. "Report of the President," in *Biennial Report of the Louisiana State Board of Health to the General Assembly of the State of Louisiana* (1914–1915): 18, LSA.

88. "Health Train Arrives; Visited by Hundreds," *Macon Daily Telegraph*, December 6, 1914.

89. Gallishoff, "Germs Know No Color Line," 28–30 and 41. On African American health activism, see Susan L. Smith, *Sick and Tired: Black Women's Health Activism in America, 1890–1950* (Philadelphia: University of Pennsylvania Press, 1995).

90. Here is a sampling: "Health Train to Tour Louisiana," *Fort Worth Star-Telegram*, November 5, 1910; in the Woman's Clubdom section, *The Anaconda Standard* (Anaconda, Montana), May 14, 1911; "Public Opinion Comment of Leading Newspapers on a Variety of Topics—The Gospel of Health," *Baltimore American*, May 29, 1911; "Exhibits Train from Louisiana on How Best to Live," *Salt Lake*

Telegram, August 7, 1911; "Louisiana Plans Unique Exhibit," *State* (Columbia, South Carolina), October 1, 1911.

91. "The A.M.A. Trip of the Louisiana Health Exhibit Car," *Southern Medical Journal* 48, no. 9 (1911): 654–56.

92. "Report of the President," in *Biennial Report of the Louisiana State Board of Health to the General Assembly of the State of Louisiana* (1910–1911): 33.

93. "News/Opinion," *Macon Daily Telegraph*, December 7, 1914.

94. "Report of the President," in *Report of the Louisiana State Board of Health* (1912–1913): 127, LSA.

95. Ibid., 129.

96. Advertisement, *The Kansas City Star*, May 20, 1914.

97. "Report of the President," in *Biennial Report of the Louisiana State Board of Health to the General Assembly of the State of Louisiana* (1914–1915): 15–16, LSA; "The Wine of Cardui Suit," *JAMA* 66, no. 12 (1916): 900; "The Case of the Chattanooga Medicine Co. against Dr. Dowling," *National Druggist* 46 (1916): 84; "Wine of Cardui Activities," *JAMA* 64 (1915): 745.

98. "Report of the President," in *Biennial Report of the Louisiana State Board of Health to the General Assembly of the State of Louisiana* (1914–1915): 15–16; "The Wine of Cardui Suit," *JAMA* 66, no. 12 (1916): 900.

99. "The Case of the Chattanooga Medicine Co. against Dr. Dowling," *National Druggist* 46 (1916): 84.

100. "What Was Found by the Chemists of the Louisiana State Board of Health," *JAMA* 70, no. 14 (1918): 1024; "Louisiana," *Southern Medical Journal* 9, no. 4 (1916): 22.

101. "Wine of Cardui Wins Suit," *New York Times*, June 23, 1916. The AMA, however, interpreted the result as vindication. See James Harvey Young, *The Medical Messiahs: A Social History of Health Quackery in Twentieth-Century America* (Princeton, NJ: Princeton University Press, 1967), 142. See also Susan Strasser, "Sponsorship and Snake Oil: Medicine Shows and Contemporary Public Culture," in *Public Culture: Diversity, Democracy, and Community in the United States*, ed. Marguerite S. Shaffer (Philadelphia: University of Philadelphia Press, 2008), 91–113.

102. The appeal of the "medicine show" continued into the mid-twentieth century, as evidenced by the popularity of the Hadacol tour of 1950. See Young, *The Medical Messiahs*, 323–24.

103. "Report of the President," in *Biennial Report of the Louisiana State Board of Health to the General Assembly of the State of Louisiana* (1914–1915): 10, LSA.

104. Ibid., 44.

105. Ibid., 47.

106. "Report of the President," in *Report of the Louisiana State Board of Health* (1912–1913): 128, LSA.

107. In 1931, Dowling died in New Orleans after "falling under the wheels of a train being ferried across the Mississippi." "Dr. Oscar Dowling Killed," *New York Times*, January 4, 1931.

108. Duffy, *The Sanitarians*, 227; see also Mike Miller, "Biography of Oscar Dowling, M.D., Montgomery, Alabama," http://files.usgwarchives.org/al/montgomery/bios/odowling.txt.

109. *State v. Dowling*, 167 La. 907, 912, https://casetext.com/case/state-v-dowling-9.

110. For a biography of Joseph Y. Porter and a positive assessment of his policies for the state of Florida, see Janice Redington Ballo, "Pointing the Way to Health: A History

of the Florida State Board of Health during the Administration of Dr. Joseph Y. Porter, 1889–1917" (master's thesis, Florida State University, 1996).

111. Joseph Y. Porter to C. J. Memminger, December 6, 1916, RG 894, Series 46, Box 31, Folder 6, State Archives of Florida, Tallahassee, Florida (hereinafter SAF).

112. Joseph Y. Porter to J. E. Taylor, November 11, 1914, RG 894, Series 46, Box 28, Folder 4, SAF.

113. State Board of Health of Florida, *Twenty-Seventh Annual Report of the State Board of Health of Florida* (1915): 24, State Library of Florida, Tallahassee (hereinafter SLF).

114. Gardner T. Swarts Jr. to Joseph Y. Porter, October 24, 1914, RG 894 Series 46, Box 28, Folder 3, SAF.

115. Gardner T. Swarts Jr. to Joseph Y. Porter, October 7, 1914, RG894 Series 46, Box 28, Folder 3, SAF.

116. Gardner T. Swarts Jr. to Joseph Y. Porter, December 2, 1914, RG 894, Series 46, Box 28, Folder 5, SAF.

117. "Interview of Friday, Dec. 10, 1914," RG 894, Series 46, Box 28, Folder 5, SAF; Joseph Y. Porter to Gardner T. Swarts Jr., October 25, 1914, RG 894, Series 46, Box 28, Folder 3, SAF; Joseph Y. Porter to Gardner T. Swarts Jr., November 6, 1914, RG 894 Series 46, Box 28, Folder 4, SAF.

118. "Florida's Health Exhibit" (Florida), *Health Notes* 10, no. 1 (1915): 3, SLF.

119. Joseph Y. Porter to Secretary, Board of Trade, Melbourne, July 17, 1915, RG 894, Series 46, Box 29, Folder 3, SAF.

120. "Florida's Health Exhibit" (Florida), *Health Notes* 10, no. 1 (1915): 3, SLF.

121. Joseph Y. Porter to W. H. Beardsley, March 22, 1915, RG 894, Series 46, Box 28, Folder 8, SAF.

122. Henry S. Marks to Joseph Y. Porter, December 24, 1914, RG 894, Series 46, Box 28, Folder 5, SAF.

123. Letter from Maurice E. Heck to Joseph Y. Porter, March 25, 1915, RG 894, Series 46, Box 28, Folder 8, SAF.

124. Joseph Y. Porter to Maurice E. Heck, March 24, 1915, RG 894, Series 46, Box 28, Folder 8, SAF.

125. "Worthy of Imitation by Other Teachers and Cities of Florida" (Florida), *Health Notes* 10, no. 4 (1915): 106, SLF.

126. Joseph Y. Porter to Frank J. Fearnside, February 17, 1915, RG 894, Series 46, Box 28, Folder 7, SAF.

127. Joseph Y. Porter to Southern Express Company, February 6, 1915, RG 894, Series 46, Box 28, Folder 7, SAF.

128. Joseph Y. Porter to W. P. Boger, July 10, 1915, RG 894, Series 46, Box 29, Folder 3, SAF.

129. Joseph Y. Porter to George A. Paddock, May 25, 1915, RG 894, Series 46, Box 29, Folder 2, SAF.

130. Joseph Y. Porter to Henry B. Marks, January 20, 1915, RG 894 Series 46, Box 28, Folder 6, SAF; Joseph Y. Porter to Warren H. Booker, June 25, 1916, RG 894, Series 46, Box 30, Folder 1, SAF.

131. Joseph Y. Porter to Warren H. Booker, June 25, 1916, RG 894, Series 46, Box 30, Folder 2, SAF. See also "Public Health Administration in Florida," *Public Health Reports* 31, no. 22 (June 1916): 1392–93, SLF, http://www.ncbi.nlm.nih.gov/pmc/articles/PMC2013665/pdf/pubhealthreporig03352-0001.pdf; "State Health Train,"

American Journal of Public Health 6, no. 6 (June 1916): 601–2, http://www.ncbi .nlm.nih.gov/pmc/articles/PMC1286881/pdf/amjphealth00094-0065.pdf.

132. U.S. Bureau of the Census, "Table 6. Urban and Rural Population, by Divisions and States: 1930 and 1920," in *Fifteenth Census of the United States, Volume 2: General Report, Statistics, and Subject* (Washington, D.C.: Government Printing Office), 10. In 1920, the majority of residents living in rural areas in Florida were white, almost 66 percent. The percentage of African Americans living in rural areas had declined since 1900, when they constituted 43 percent of the state's rural population, to 34 percent in 1920. U.S. Bureau of the Census, "Florida: Table 1. Color or Race, Nativity, Percentage, and Sex for the State and Urban and Rural Population: 1920, 1910, and 1900," in *Fourteenth Census of the United States Taken in the Year 1920, Volume 3: Population 1920: Composition and Characteristics of the Population by States* (Washington, D.C.: Government Printing Office), 184. This drop in percentage is evidence of the number of African Americans who chose to leave the South during this time in search of better opportunities. On the Great Migration, see James Grossman, *Land of Hope: Chicago, Black Southerners, and the Great Migration* (Chicago: University of Chicago Press, 1989).

133. Florida's mill system of taxation provided the Florida State Board of Health a steady income upon which to conduct activities. Florida also empowered its board of health to "make and promulgate a sanitary code carrying the weight of the law." Ettling, *The Germ of Laziness*, 119.

134. Joseph Y. Porter to Oscar Dowling, March 25, 1915, RG 894, Series 46, Box 28, Folder 8, SAF.

135. Asst to General Manager to Joseph Y. Porter, March 16, 1915, RG 894, Series 46, Box 28, Folder 8, SAF.

136. The bill that failed to pass was about the board's funding.

137. (Florida) *Health Notes* 10, no. 6 (1915): back cover, SLF.

138. (Florida) *Health Notes* 10, no. 7 (1915): 207, SLF.

139. "Roast for B. of H.," *Free Press*, August 24, 1916, RG 894, Series 46, Box 31, Folder 5, SAF.

140. "A National Clearing-House for Social Surveys and Exhibits," *Survey* (October 5, 1912), Series 3, Box 33, Folder 264, Russell Sage Foundation, RAC.

141. E. G. Routzahn to Joseph Y. Porter, January 5, 1915, RG 894, Series 46, Box 28, Folder 6, SAF; E. G. Routzahn to Joseph Y. Porter, September 21, 1915, RG 894, Series 46, Box 29, Folder 4, SAF.

142. "Florida's 'Health Train,'" *Health Notes* 11, no. 1 (1916): 419, SLF.

143. Clipping from *Free Press*, November 13, 1916, State Board of Health Correspondence, RG 894, Series 46, Box 31, Folder, 5, SAF.

144. "Eden Musee Faces Bankruptcy Court," *New York Times*, June 8, 1915.

145. Richard Hargrave to Joseph Y. Porter, October 5, 1916, RG 894, Series 46, Box 31, Folder, 4, SAF.

146. Clipping from *Bradford County Times*, November 13, 1916, RG 894, Series 46, Box 31, Folder, 5, SAF.

147. Joseph Y. Porter to Avery G. Powell, November 13, 1916, RG 894, Series 46, Box 31, Folder, 5, SAF.

148. "Public Health Administration in Florida," *Public Health Reports* 31, no. 22 (June 1916): 1392, http://www.ncbi.nlm.nih.gov/pmc/articles/PMC2013665/pdf/pubhealth reporig03352-0001.pdf.

149. Ibid., 1375.

150. Mrs. F. A. Scott to Joseph Y. Porter, November 11, 1916, RG 894, Series 46, Box 31, Folder 5, SAF.

151. Frank J. Fearnside to Joseph Y. Porter, January 19, 1916, RG894, Series 900, Box 3, Folder 40, SAF.

152. C. J. Memminger to Joseph Y. Porter, December 19, 1916, RG 894, Series 46, Box 31, Folder 6, SAF.

153. Joseph Y. Porter to Mr. Swanson, December 2, 1916, RG 894, Series 46, Box 31, Folder 6, SAF.

154. Joseph Y. Porter to Mr. Swanson, December 2, 1916, RG 894, Series 46, Box 31, Folder 6, SAF.

155. Ibid.

156. C. J. Memminger to Joseph Y. Porter, December 19, 1916, RG 894, Series 46, Box 31, Folder 6, SAF.

157. Although he was seventy years old, Porter resigned so that he could serve in the U.S. Army as a medical officer during World War I. He did not return once the war concluded, perhaps because he and the new governor, Sidney J. Catts, "saw little in the same light." Albert V. Hardy and May Pynchon, *Milestones and Milestones: Florida's Public Health from 1889* (Jacksonville: Florida State Board of Health, 1964), 28–31.

158. Hardy and Pynchon, *Milestones and Milestones*, 28–31.

159. W. H. Cox to C. H. Clair Drake, January 3, 1918, RG 894, Series 46, Box 32, Folder 4, SAF; C. H. Clair Drake to W. H. Cox, January 10, 1918, RG 894, Series 46, Box 32, Folder 4, SAF.

160. Graham to Miss Doris H. Hurnie, August 18, 1958, RG 894, Series 900, Box 3, Folder 40, SAF.

4. Controversial Exhibits

1. Mike Wallace, *Mickey Mouse History and Other Essays on American Memory* (Philadelphia: Temple University Press, 1996), especially chapters Museums and Controversy and The Battle of the *Enola Gay*; Edward T. Linenthal and Tom Engelhardt, *History Wars: The Enola Gay and Other Battles for the American Past* (New York: Henry Holt and Company, 1996); Steven C. Dubin, *Displays of Power: Controversy in the American Museum from the Enola Gay to Sensation* (New York: New York University Press, 1999); James Oliver Horton and Lois E. Horton, *Slavery and Public History: The Tough Stuff of American History* (Chapel Hill: North Carolina University Press, 2006).

2. Plastination is a process of replacing body fat and water with plastics. Elena Canadelli, "'Scientific Peep Show': The Human Body in Contemporary Science Museums," *Nuncius* 26 (2011): 166. On the history of "body" exhibits, see Erin McLeary and Elizabeth Toon, "Here Man Learns about Himself," *American Journal of Public Health* 102, no. 7 (July 2012); Klaus Vogel, "The Transparent Man—Some Comments on the History of a Symbol," in *Manifesting Medicine: Bodies and Machines*, ed. Robert Bud, Bernard Finn, and Helmuth Trischler (Amsterdam: Harwood Academic, 1999).

3. Andrew Martinez, "A Mixed Reception for Modernism: The 1913 Armory Show at the Chicago Art Institute of Chicago," *Art Institute of Chicago Museum Studies* 19, no. 1 (1993): 31–58.

4. A brief discussion about the rejection of the exhibit appears in the introduction to James V. Costanzo Sr., *New Neighbors, Old Friends: Morristown's Italian Community, 1880–1924* (Morristown, NJ: Morris County Historical Society, 1982), vii.

5. Alan M. Kraut, *Silent Travelers: Germs, Genes, and the Immigrant Menace* (Baltimore: Johns Hopkins University Press, 1994), especially chap. 5.

6. Donna Gabaccia, *From Sicily to Elizabeth Street: Housing and Social Change among Italian Immigrants, 1880–1930* (Albany: State University of New York Press, 1984); Diane C. Vecchio, *Merchants, Midwives, and Laboring Women: Italian Migrants in Urban America* (Urbana: University of Illinois Press, 2006), especially chap. 4.

7. Bureau of Industrial Statistics of New Jersey, *The Industrial Directory of New Jersey* (Camden, NJ: S. Chew & Sons. Co., 1915), 331.

8. Ibid.

9. Ibid., 331–32.

10. Ibid., 331.

11. Bureau of Industrial Statistics, Department of Labor, *The Industrial Directory of New Jersey* (Paterson, NJ: New Printing Company, 1918), 375–76.

12. Ibid., 331–32; Bureau of Industrial Statistics, Department of Labor, *The Industrial Directory of New Jersey* (Paterson, NJ: New Printing Company, 1918), 375–76.

13. Federal Writers' Project, *New Jersey: A Guide to Its Present and Past* (New York: Viking, 1939), 284–85.

14. Costanzo, *New Neighbors, Old Friends*, 84.

15. Ibid., 67.

16. Ibid., 82.

17. Report of the Social and Religious Survey of Morristown, New Jersey, 1914: 10 and 45–46; HM6 Pres, North Jersey History & Genealogy Center, Morristown, NJ (hereinafter NJHGC). On women's shifting opinions as to the desirability of domestic service at the turn of the twentieth century, especially based on ethnicity and race, see Joanne Meyerowitz, *Women Adrift: Independent Wage Earners in Chicago, 1880–1930* (Chicago: University of Chicago Press, 1988).

18. U.S. Bureau of the Census, *Reports by States with Statistics for Counties, Cities, and Other Civil Divisions* (Washington, D.C.: GPO, 1910); *Volume 3: Population*, New Jersey, Table III: Composition and Characteristics of the Population for Places of 10,000 to 25,000, 147, https://www2.census.gov/library/publications/decennial /1910/volume-3/volume-3-p2.pdf.

19. Some of Morristown's African American citizens traced their roots back to slavery. Others migrated to find work in the brickyards. See information regarding African Americans and Morristown in *Historical Summaries of Neighborhood House* (1940), HM 513 MSS, Box 9, Folder 5, NJHGC.

20. Bureau of Industrial Statistics of New Jersey, *The Industrial Directory of New Jersey* (Camden, NJ: S. Chew & Sons. Co., 1915), 331. In 1910, the U.S. Census enumerated 185 people with Russian heritage (107 born in Russia, 78 with at least one Russian parent). It enumerated only six people as being from Greece.

21. "Morristown Italians Growing Prosperous," *Newark Sunday Call*, July 14, 1907.

22. Ibid.

23. Costanzo, *New Neighbors, Old Friends*, 15, 82.

24. "History of Neighborhood House," HM 513 MSS, Box 9, Folder 5, NJHGC.

25. Ibid.

26. Ibid.

27. Ibid.

28. On the history of the settlement house movement in various forms, including religious, see Ruth Crocker, *Social Work and Social Order: The Settlement Movement in Two Industrial Cities, 1889–1930* (Urbana: University of Illinois Press, 1992);

Allen F. Davis, *Spearheads for Reform: The Social Settlements and the Progressive Movement, 1890–1914* (Oxford: Oxford University Press, 1967); Maureen Flanagan, *Seeing with Their Hearts: Chicago Women and the Vision of the Good City, 1871– 1933* (Princeton, NJ: Princeton University Press, 2002); Deirdre Moloney, *American Catholic Lay Groups and Transatlantic Social Reform in the Progressive Era* (Chapel Hill: University of North Carolina Press, 2002); Robyn Muncy, *Creating a Female Dominion in American Reform, 1890–1935* (Oxford: Oxford University Press, 1994).

29. Report for 1914–1915, Annual Reports Neighborhood House 1913–, HM 513 MSS, Box 1, Folder 21, NJHGC.

30. Report of Italian Settlement House, from November 30 to January 1, 1908, Monthly Report of the Neighborhood House 1905–1908, HM 513 MSS, Box 1, Folder 2, NJHGC.

31. Ibid.

32. Ibid.

33. Ibid.

34. Costanzo, *New Neighbors, Old Friends*, 120–24.

35. *Minutes of the General Assembly of the Presbyterian Church in the United States of America* XIV (August 1914): 375, NJHGC.

36. Ibid., 375; Report of the Social and Religious Survey of Morristown, New Jersey, 1914; HM6 Pres, NJHGC.

37. I made this determination by analyzing the surnames of the students. The overwhelming majority had English surnames. Drew University, *Annual Catalogue* (1913–1914), https://hdl.handle.net/2027/uiug.30112111548308.

38. Report of the Social and Religious Survey of Morristown, New Jersey, 1914; HM6 Pres, NJHGC.

39. Ibid.

40. Ibid.

41. Ibid., 11.

42. Ibid., 22.

43. Ibid., 25.

44. Ibid., 30.

45. Ibid., 32–33.

46. Ibid. Unfortunately, no archival copy of the exhibit materials appears to have been preserved.

47. "Social Service Exhibit," *Morris County Chronicle*, March 10, 1914.

48. *Minutes of the General Assembly of the Presbyterian Church in the United States of America* XIV (August 1914): 375, NJHGC.

49. "Stelzle's Ideas on Town's Needs," *Morris County Chronicle*, March 10, 1914.

50. "Health Board at Issue with Survey," *Morris County Chronicle*, March 10, 1914. Glazebrook was the secretary of the board of health. "Tells Reason for High Rate," *Daily Record*, March 10, 1914.

51. "Smashing of the Morristown Survey Exhibit," *Survey* 32, no. 1 (1914): 4.

52. "Health Board at Issue with Survey," *Morris County Chronicle*, March 10, 1914.

53. *N.E.A. Bulletin* 6–7, no. 1 (September 1917): 233; Kendrick Charles Babcock, "Accredited Secondary Schools in the United States," *United States Bureau of Education Bulletin* no. 29 (1913): 44.

54. "Morristown," *Newark Sunday Call*, September 14, 1913; "Morristown Votes on High School," *Newark Sunday Call*, July 19, 1914.

55. "Health Board at Issue with Survey," *Morris County Chronicle*, March 10, 1914.

56. "Tells Reasons for High Rate," *Daily Record*, March 10, 1914.

57. "Social Uplift Show Wrecked in New Jersey," *New York Times*, March 13, 1914.

58. "Negro School Closed Half Century Ago," *Morristown Daily Record*, September 26, 1936, Morris School District Records, HM5 MSS MSD, Series 1, Box 11, Folder 12, NJHGC.

59. "Background," Historical Summaries of Neighborhood House (1940), HM 513 MSS, Box 9, Folder 5, NJHGC.

60. Hannibal Gerald Duncan, "The Changing Race Relationship in the Border and Northern States," PhD thesis (Philadelphia: University of Pennsylvania, 1922), 38. Marion M. Thompson found similar issues that perpetuated segregation. Marion M. Thompson Wright, *The Education of Negroes in New Jersey* (New York: Bureau of Publications, Teachers College, Columbia University, New York, 1941), 197–98, Morris School District Records, HM5 MSS MSD, Series 1, Box 11, Folder 12, NJHGC.

61. "Social Uplift Show Wrecked in New Jersey," *New York Times*, March 13, 1914.

62. "Citizens Protest against Survey," *Morris County Chronicle*, March 17, 1914; "Italians Resent Reflections with Raid," *Washington Times*, March 13, 1914.

63. "Italians Raid Survey Exhibit: Throng Visits Public School," *Daily Record*, March 12, 1914.

64. Ibid.

65. Some of the newspaper coverage inverts these events. It is my conclusion that because the police were called in to disperse the crowd and quell the disturbance at the exhibit, it is more reasonable to believe that the group first went to see Wiley, became impatient, turned around the corner, and attacked the exhibit. Regarding the estimated number, see "Italians Raid Survey Exhibit: Throng Visits Public School," *Daily Record*, March 12, 1914.

66. "A Surprise for the Uplifters," *New York Times*, March 14, 1914.

67. "Morristown, N.J., March 12," *Bulletin of Photography* (March 1914): 346.

68. "Pellegrin Venezia," 1910 United States Federal Census Manuscript. Accessed via Ancestry.com.

69. *Morristown City Directory*, 1912 and 1913, NJHGC.

70. "Citizens Protest against Survey," *Morris County Chronicle*, March 17, 1914. Merrill Morris was eighteen years old. In the 1910 U.S. Census, he was listed as living with his aunt, Lydia Morris, and his siblings. His aunt owned the Morris Art Store, which was located at 74 Elm Street in 1914 according to the city directory. Accessed via ancestry.com. I have not found any additional information that would indicate why Morris was put in charge of watching over the exhibit.

71. "Citizens Protest against Survey," *Morris County Chronicle*, March 17, 1914; "Social Uplift Show Wrecked in New Jersey," *New York Times*, March 13, 1914; "Italians Mob Uplift Show," *Washington Herald*, March 13, 1914.

72. "Italians Raid Survey Exhibit: Throng Visits Public School," *Daily Record*, March 12, 1914; "Citizens Protest against Survey," *Morris County Chronicle*, March 17, 1914.

73. "Italians Raid Survey Exhibit: Throng Visits Public School," *Daily Record*, March 12, 1914.

74. *Morristown City Directory*, 1912 and 1913, NJHGC.

75. "Fedele Lucia," 1920 United States Federal Census Manuscript. Accessed via Ancestry.com. "Corvine Verillo," 1910 United States Federal Census Manuscript. Accessed via Ancestry.com. "Pellegrin Venezia," 1910 United States Federal Census Manuscript. Accessed via Ancestry.com.

76. *Morristown City Directory*, 1912 and 1913, NJHGC.
77. "The Social Survey," *Morris County Chronicle*, March 17, 1914.
78. "Is Morristown Really Decading?" *Morris County Chronicle*, March 17, 1914; "Speakers for the Exhibit," *Daily Record*, March 14, 1914.
79. "Is Morristown Really Decading?" *Morris County Chronicle*, March 17, 1914.
80. "Citizens Protest against Survey," *Morris County Chronicle*, March 17, 1914.
81. Ibid.
82. *Daily Record*, March 11, 1914.
83. "Citizens Protest against Survey," *Morris County Chronicle*, March 17, 1914.
84. "Social Survey Sponsors Explain," *Morris County Chronicle*, March 17, 1914.
85. "Close of the Social Survey," *Daily Record*, March 13, 1914.
86. Ibid.
87. "Italians Destroy Pictures," *Tulsa Daily World*, March 13, 1914; "Uplift without Understanding," *Boston Evening Transcript*, March 14, 1914; "Uplift Jarred by Italians," *Los Angeles Times*, March 13, 1914.
88. "Uplift without Understanding," *New York Tribune*, March 13, 1914.
89. "The Morristown Survey: Not Intended to Put Poor Foreigners to Shame," *New York Times*, March 18, 1914.
90. "Smashing of the Morristown Survey Exhibit," *Survey* 32, no. 1 (1914): 4.
91. Ibid., 5.
92. Ibid.
93. Ibid., 4–5.
94. "Violation of Ethics?" *Jerseyman*, March 20, 1914.
95. Ibid.
96. "Health Board at Issue with Survey," *Morris County Chronicle*, March 10, 1914.
97. "Plan Tuberculosis Exhibit," *Morris County Chronicle*, March 10, 1914; "Tuberculosis Exhibit Opens," *Daily Record*, March 17, 1914.
98. "Gives Talks to the Italians," *Daily Record*, March 19, 1914.
99. "Speakers for the Exhibit," *Daily Record*, March 14, 1914.
100. "Exhibit Closed after 5 Days," *Daily Record*, March 21, 1914.
101. For a brief discussion of this event, see Kathleen A. Tobin, *The American Religious Debate over Birth Control, 1907–1937* (Jefferson, NC: McFarland, 2001), 125.
102. On the history of the birth control movement in the United States, see Linda Gordon, *The Moral Property of Women: A History of Birth Control in America* (Urbana: University of Illinois Press, 2002); Carole R. McCann, *Birth Control Politics in the United States, 1916–1945* (Ithaca, NY: Cornell University Press, 1994). Sanger resigned from the ABCL in the summer of 1928, after the events in New York. Sanger and those who followed her believed that changing federal laws that stymied people's access should be the organization's foremost priority. She also continued to think that controversy helped to move the movement forward. Eleanor Jones, ABCL's new leader, disagreed. She wanted to focus on creating clinics, and she moved to ally with the American Eugenics Society. To say that the role of eugenics in Sanger, Jones, and other proponents' beliefs about birth control was complicated is an understatement. Ideas about "fit" and "unfit" and whether those conditions were controlled by heredity, environment, or a combination left room for debate as to who should be the target audience for birth control. See McCann, *Birth Control Politics*, 177–82. Those differing ideas do not seem to have been an issue over the ABCL's proposed display at the exhibition.

103. Cathy Moran Hajo, *Birth Control on Main Street: Organizing Clinics in the United States, 1916–1939* (Urbana: University of Illinois Press, 2010), chaps. 1 and 2. While providing contraception was officially only supposed to go to married women, single women found ways to get through the door. Hajo, *Birth Control on Main Street*, 54.

104. Manon Parry, *Broadcasting Birth Control: Mass Media and Family Planning* (New Brunswick, NJ: Rutgers University Press, 2013), especially chap. 2.

105. "Exposition for Parents Is a Many-Sided Show," *New York Times*, April 22, 1928.

106. "Parents' Exposition," *Hygeia* 6, no. 5 (May 1928): 296.

107. Annual Report of the President, U.P.A., 1926–27, Board of Education Records, Series 911, United Parents Association, 1921–1989, Subseries 1, Box 1, Folder 1, New York Municipal Archives (hereinafter NYMA).

108. "Parents of Pupils in 50 Schools Meet," *New York Times*, May 7, 1922.

109. Typewritten notes 1921–1925, n.d., Series 911, United Parents Association, 1921–1989, Subseries 1, Box 1, Folder 1, NYMA.

110. Annual Report of the President, U.P.A., 1926–27, Board of Education Records, Series 911, United Parents Association, 1921–1989, Subseries 1, Box 1, Folder 1, NYMA.

111. Evaluation Report of the Parents' Exposition, n.d., Board of Education Records, Series 911, United Parents Association, 1921–1989, Subseries 4.1, Box 8, Folder 14, NYMA.

112. Ibid.

113. "A Great New Building," *New York Times*, February 27, 1893; "New Grand Central Palace," *New York Times*, May 20, 1911.

114. "Parents' Exposition Opened by Walker," *New York Times*, April 22, 1928.

115. Display Ad 187, *New York Times*, April 25, 1928.

116. "Parent's Exposition," *Journal of Social Hygiene* 14, no. 3 (1928): 174. Ernst was married to Bernard M. L. Ernst, who was best known for his friendship and business relationship with Harry Houdini. After Houdini's death, Ernst succeeded him as president of the Society of American Magicians. "Mrs. Bernard Ernst," *New York Times*, July 25, 1972.

117. "New York City's Parents' Exposition," *Home Economist* 6, no. 3 (March 1928): 57.

118. Ibid.

119. "Radio Talks to Aid Parents Exposition," *New York Times*, March 24, 1928.

120. "Plans for Parents Exposition," *New York Times*, March 11, 1928.

121. "An Exposition for Parents," *New York Times*, March 4, 1928.

122. "Exposition for Parents Is a Many-Sided Show," *New York Times*, April 22, 1928.

123. "Parents Exposition Viewed by 250,000," *New York Times*, April 29, 1928.

124. "Plan Living Room Exhibit," *New York Times*, April 15, 1928; "Exposition for Parents Is a Many-Sided Show," *New York Times*, April 22, 1928.

125. "Exposition for Parents Is a Many-Sided Show," *New York Times*, April 22, 1928.

126. Program, Parents' Exposition, Board of Education Records, Series 911, United Parents Association, 1921–1989, Subseries 2.1, Box 2, Folder 7, NYMA.

127. "Exposition for Parents Is a Many-Sided Show," *New York Times*, April 22, 1928.

128. Evaluation Report of the Parents' Exposition, n.d., Board of Education Records, Series 911, United Parents Association, 1921–1989, Subseries 4.1, Box 8, Folder 14, NYMA. The second time a similar exposition was held, the Board of Estimates paid $35,000 for the Board of Education's share of the rent for exhibit space. Report to Board of Governors From: Executive Secretary on Progress of Work from June 1 to

November 1, 1928, Board of Education Records, Series 911, United Parents Association, 1921–1989, Subseries 4.1, Box 8, Folder 4, NYMA.

129. "The Parents' Exposition," *New York Times*, April 26, 1928.

130. "Parents Exposition Viewed by 250,000," *New York Times*, April 29, 1928.

131. "An Exposition for Parents," *New York Times*, March 4, 1928; "Exposition for Parents Is a Many-Sided Show," *New York Times*, April 22, 1928.

132. Program, Parents' Exposition, Board of Education Records, Series 911, United Parents Association, 1921–1989, Subseries 2.1, Box 2, Folder 17, NYMA. Published by the American Social Hygiene Association in 1928, Torrey's brief book described work at three Oregon schools that introduced biology into their elementary curriculum. Students learned about reproduction in flora and fauna and, for more advanced children, issues of human physiology.

133. Program, Parents' Exposition, Board of Education Records, Series 911, United Parents Association, 1921–1989, Subseries 2.1, Box 2, Folder 17, NYMA. Answering Children's Questions: Sex Education was a thirteen-page pamphlet printed by the Child Study Association of America in 1925.

134. Margaret Sanger, *Birth Control Refused Space at Parent's Exposition*, April 1928. Typed draft article. Source: *Margaret Sanger Papers*, Library of Congress, LCM 129:55, http://www.nyu.edu/projects/sanger/webedition/app/documents/show.php?sanger Doc=128018.xml.

135. "Parents' Exposition Opened by Walker," *New York Times*, April 22, 1928.

136. Unfortunately, no archival evidence about what exactly the ABCL was going to display seems to exist.

137. "School Show Bars Birth Control Body," *New York Times*, April 20, 1928.

138. "Birth Control Body Fights School Ban," *New York Times*, April 21, 1928.

139. Ibid.

140. Ibid.

141. "Parents' Exposition Opened by Walker," *New York Times*, April·22, 1928.

142. Program, Parents' Exposition, Board of Education Records, Series 911, United Parents Association, 1921–1989, Subseries 2.1, Box 2, Folder 17, NYMA.

143. "Birth Control Body Fights School Ban," *New York Times*, April 21, 1928.

144. Ibid.

145. On the history of how the birth control movement used mass media, see Manon Parry, *Broadcasting Birth Control: Mass Media and Family Planning* (New Brunswick, NJ: Rutgers University Press, 2013).

146. "Birth Control Ban Arouses Protests," *New York Times*, April 24, 1928.

147. Ibid. It does not appear that Bruno Lasker was related to Albert Lasker, a contemporary and philanthropist of medicine, particularly of cancer.

148. "Parents," *Time* 11, no. 19 (May 7, 1928): 36–37.

149. "Birth Control Ban Arouses Protests," *New York Times*, April 24, 1928.

150. Margaret Sanger, *Birth Control Refused Space at Parent's Exposition*.

151. McCann, *Birth Control Politics*, 68–69.

152. "To Vote on Birth Control Laws," *New York Times*, January 4, 1928.

153. "Women's City Club for Birth Control," *New York Times*, January 5, 1928.

154. "Catholic Women Hit Birth Control," *New York Times*, January 14, 1928.

155. "Editorial," *Birth Control Review* XII, no. 5 (May 1928): 137.

156. "Mrs. Sanger Calls Catholics Bigots," *New York Times*, April 25, 1928.

157. "It Seems to Heywood Broun," *Nation* 126 (May 9, 1928): 532.

158. "New York," *Birth Control Review* XII, no. 6 (June 1928): 189.

159. "News Notes: United States: New York," *Birth Control Review* 12, no. 11 (November 1928): 324–25.

160. Agenda, Governing Board, June 13, 1929, Board of Education Records, Series 911, United Parents Association, 1921–1989, Subseries 4.1, Box 8, Folder 5, NYMA.

161. Minutes, Governing Board, United Parents' Associations, June 13, 1929, Board of Education Records, Series 911, United Parents Association, 1921–1989, Subseries 4.1, Box 8, Folder 5, NYMA.

162. Minutes, Governing Board, United Parents' Associations, September 26, 1929, Board of Education Records, Series 911, United Parents Association, 1921–1989, Subseries 4.1, Box 8, Folder 5, NYMA.

163. Agenda, Governing Board, United Parents' Associations, October 24, 1929, November 27, 1929, and December 19, 1929, Board of Education Records, Series 911, United Parents Association, 1921–1989, Subseries 4.1, Box 8, Folder 5, NYMA.

164. Minutes, Governing Board, December 18, 1929, Board of Education Records, Series 911, United Parents Association, 1921–1989, Subseries 4.1, Box 8, Folder 5, NYMA.

165. Ibid.

166. Ibid.

167. Evaluation Report of the Parents' Exposition, n.d., Board of Education Records, Series 911, United Parents Association, 1921–1989, Subseries 4.1, Box 8, Folder 14, NYMA.

168. 1921–1925, n.d., Board of Education Records, Series 911, United Parents Association, 1921–1989, Subseries 2.1, Box 2, Folder 3, NYMA. Although the handwriting on the front page of these notes is 1921–1925, the information extends into the 1930s.

169. Evaluation Report of the Parents' Exposition, n.d., Board of Education Records, Series 911, United Parents Association, 1921–1989, Subseries 4.1, Box 8, Folder 14, NYMA.

Conclusion

1. Holmer N. Calver, "Marking Mass Education," *American Journal of Public Health* 22, no. 1 (January 1932): 55. This was a reprint of Calver's talk before the American Public Health Association's annual meeting.

2. Calver, "Marking Mass Education," 56.

3. Erin McLeary and Elizabeth Toon, "'Here Man Learns about Himself': Visual Education and the Rise and Fall of the American Museum of Health," *American Journal of Public Health* 102, no. 7 (July 2012): e27–e36.

4. Ibid., e34.

5. Bruno Gebhard, "Health Museums in the United States: Review and Outlook," *Curator* 8, no. 2 (1965): 144–45.

6. Ibid., 144.

7. Ibid., 160.

8. Ibid., 146.

9. Ibid.

Index

Note: An "f" after a page number indicates a figure.

Torrey, Harry Beal, 93

Train exhibits. *See* Health trains

Traveling exhibits and shows: on child welfare, 27–29; in health trains, 8, 52–74; limitations of films in, 6; on tuberculosis, 14–15, 17, 18, 23, 46, 47, 53

Treichler, Paula A., 5

Tuberculosis, 7; films on, 5; mortality from, 12, 55; prevention efforts, 3–4, 12–13, 17; spread from rural to urban areas, 53, 54

Tuberculosis exhibits, 9, 12, 13–19, 30; advertising on, 18, 19f; at American Museum of Natural History, 13–14, 17–18, 53; attendance at, 14, 15, 17, 18; on California Sanitation Car, 55, 56, 59f; in Chicago, 15; children attending, 16; on child welfare, 26; community outreach in, 16; as complementary to lectures and leaflets, 16; contrast rooms in, 16; effectiveness of, 18; on Florida health train, 70; funding of, 14, 17; on industrial safety, 26; influence of, 5, 22–23; on Louisiana health train, 64; in Maryland, 17, 107n16; in Minneapolis, 15–16; in New Jersey, 88, 89; in New York City, 13–14, 17–18, 19f; in Philadelphia, 14–15; Routzahn on value of, 46; in Saint Louis World's Fair, 107n16; in settlement houses, 15, 107–108n29; Swarts models for, 45; traveling, 14–15, 17, 18, 23, 46, 47, 53; in urban planning exhibits, 13, 20, 22; visitor reaction to, 16; in Washington D.C., 17

Tulane University, and Louisiana health train, 63–64

Twenty-second Regiment Armory (NYC), City Planning Exhibition at, 21

Typhoid fever, 70–71; California Sanitation Car exhibit on, 55; spread from rural to urban areas, 53, 54

United Parents' Association of Greater New York Schools: founding of, 90; mission of, 90; Parents' Exposition of (1928), 89–97, 98; Parents' Exposition of (1929), 97; Simon as president of, 90, 91, 92–93, 94

University of Pennsylvania tuberculosis exhibit, 14

Urban planning exhibits, 7, 13, 20–22; in Chicago, 20; on industrial safety, 26; limitations of, 21; in New York City, 20–21, 22; in Pittsburgh, 22; on taxation, 21, 22; tuberculosis information in, 13, 20, 22

Venecio, Pellegrino, 85

Venereal disease films, 5

Verilli, Carmine, 85–86

Vigilante, Rose, 77

Visitor reactions: to American Birth Control League exhibits, 93–94, 96; to child welfare exhibits, 27, 28–29, 111n131; to Florida health train exhibits, 70; to industrial safety exhibits, 25; to Louisiana health train exhibits, 64; to Morristown NJ exhibits, 76, 78, 83, 85–87, 89, 98; to Rauer models, 38; to tuberculosis exhibits, 16, 89

Volker, William, 28

Washington D.C. tuberculosis exhibit, 17

White, Gaylord, 16

Wiley, J. Burton, 83–85, 88, 89

William II, Emperor of Germany, 33

Wine of Cardui elixir, 66, 126n101

Wisconsin: tuberculosis exhibit in, 15; urban planning exhibit in, 22

Wisconsin Anti-Tuberculosis Association, 46

Woman's City Club, 28

Women: bias of reformers towards, 4; birth control for, 89–90, 95; child welfare exhibits organized by, 26–27; employment of, in Morristown NJ, 77–78, 130n17; hygiene measures marketed to, 4, 103n4; low wages paid to, 28; protective legislation on, 11, 106n2; as target audience, 11f

Women's Activities Exhibit, 96

Women's Arts and Industries Exhibition, 93

Women's City Club, 95

Working class: bias of reformers towards, 4; as target audience, 9, 30, 49

World's fairs and expositions, 4–5; in New York, Hall of Man at, 99–100; in Saint Louis (*See* Saint Louis World's Exposition)

World War I, 37

Yellow fever, 1, 4

Yiddish, 15, 18, 19f

About the Author

Jennifer Lisa Koslow is an associate professor of history and director of the Historical Administration and Public History program at Florida State University. She is the author of *Cultivating Health: Los Angeles Women and Public Health Reform.*

Available titles in the Critical Issues in Health and Medicine series: